crunch time
cookbook

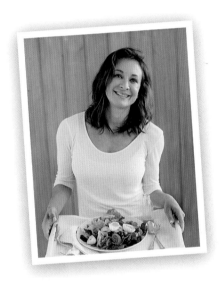

Michelle Bridges has worked in the fitness industry for
over two decades as a professional trainer and group fitness
instructor both in Australia and overseas. Her role as a trainer
on Channel Ten's *The Biggest Loser* has made her Australia's most
recognised personal trainer. She is also the author of *Crunch Time:
Lose Weight Fast and Keep It Off*, *Losing the Last Five Kilos*, *Michelle
Bridges: 5 Minutes a Day* and *The No Excuses Cookbook*.

michellebridges.com.au

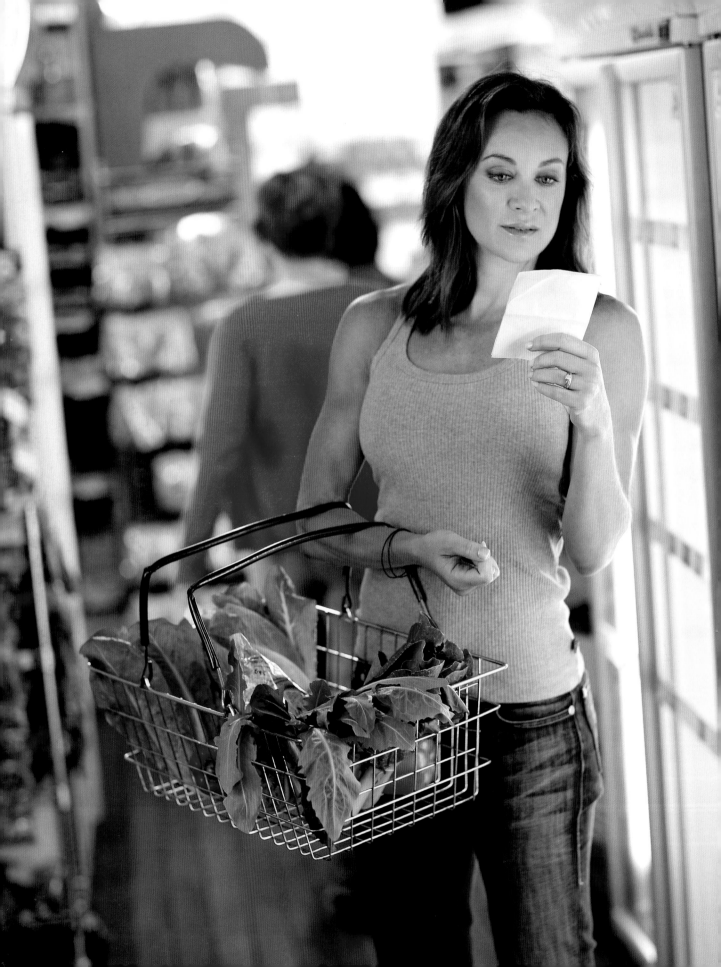

crunch time
cookbook

100 knockout recipes for rapid weight loss

michelle bridges

VIKING
an imprint of
PENGUIN BOOKS

VIKING

Published by the Penguin Group
Penguin Group (Australia)
707 Collins Street, Melbourne, Victoria 3008, Australia
(a division of Pearson Australia Group Pty Ltd)
Penguin Group (USA) Inc.
375 Hudson Street, New York, New York 10014, USA
Penguin Group (Canada)
90 Eglinton Avenue East, Suite 700, Toronto, Canada ON M4P 2Y3
(a division of Pearson Penguin Canada Inc.)
Penguin Books Ltd
80 Strand, London WC2R 0RL, England
Penguin Ireland
25 St Stephen's Green, Dublin 2, Ireland
(a division of Penguin Books Ltd)
Penguin Books India Pvt Ltd
11 Community Centre, Panchsheel Park, New Delhi – 110 017, India
Penguin Group (NZ)
67 Apollo Drive, Rosedale, North Shore 0632, New Zealand
(a division of Pearson New Zealand Ltd)
Penguin Books (South Africa) (Pty) Ltd
Rosebank Office Park, Block D, 181 Jan Smuts Avenue, Parktown North,
Johannesburg 2196, South Africa

Penguin Books Ltd, Registered Offices: 80 Strand, London WC2R 0RL, England

First published by Penguin Group (Australia), 2010

10 9

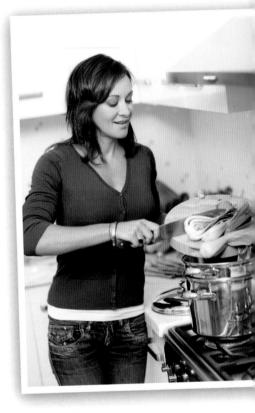

Text copyright © Michelle Bridges 2010
Photography copyright © Mark O'Meara and Nick Wilson 2010

The moral right of the author has been asserted

Design by Cameron Midson © Penguin Group (Australia)
Cover photographs by Nick Wilson and Mark O'Meara
Photography by Mark O'Meara and Nick Wilson
Styling by Michelle Noerianto
Food preparation by Jennifer Tolhurst
Food consultant Lucy Nunes
Typeset in Chaparral Pro and Vectora LH by Post Pre-press Group, Brisbane, Queensland
Colour reproduction by Splitting Image, Clayton, Victoria
Printed and bound in China by South China Printing Company

National Library of Australia
Cataloguing-in-Publication data:

Bridges, Michelle.
Crunch time cookbook/Michelle Bridges.
9780670074105 (pbk.)
Includes index.
Reducing diets – Recipes.

641.563

penguin.com.au

Contents

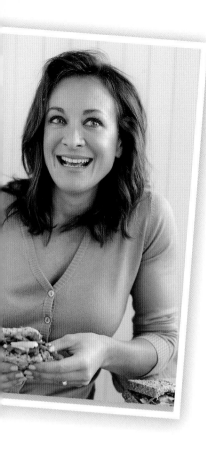

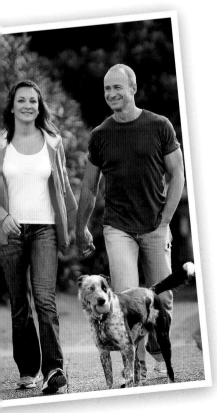

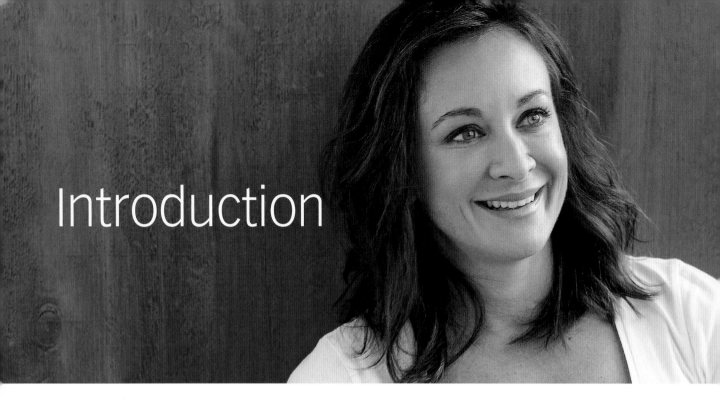

Introduction

Since I first began working in the fitness industry many years ago, I've had day-to-day contact with all kinds of people: from super-fit instructors, to overweight teenagers, to mums trying to shift the baby weight. And if there's one thing I've learnt from all this experience it's that when it comes to weight management and better health, *food is more important than exercise*. Don't get me wrong. Exercise is the fountain of youth. Drink from it daily and you will reap the most amazing benefits physically and mentally. Plus, if you are out to lose some weight, exercise will vastly accelerate the process. However, if you are exercising daily but still eating poorly or simply eating too much (whether it's nutritious or not), you could be taking one step forward and two steps back. You may have heard people say that weight loss is 70 per cent diet and 30 per cent exercise, and they're not wrong.

After another incredible season as a trainer on *The Biggest Loser*, I am even more convinced of how crucial it is to take charge of what you eat. Exercise is brilliant for building muscle tone, which pumps your metabolism and helps you burn calories even faster, but ultimately it's what you chew and swallow that gets you where you are – and to where you want to be. We all saw that the real successes on the show came from eating more nutritious food and less of it.

If I had two clients, one of whom refused to eat well and ate whatever she liked whenever she liked, but I trained her like a demon every day, and another who did no exercise but tidied up her diet so that she had a weekly calorie deficit, the non-exerciser would lose the most weight.

I'm guessing that like many people you want to be fitter and lighter than you are right now.

I'm here to tell you that the only way you are going to accelerate yourself to lean and mean is if you put in some time in the kitchen. Taking responsibility for your own nutrition is an important step towards taking responsibility for your own body and breaking the old habits that keep you stuck in a holding pattern. For those of you who already cook, you know how easy it can be. For those of you with 'L' plates, I want you to know that I am only interested in simple recipes with fresh ingredients that are quick to prepare and don't burn a hole in your budget.

At this point I have to be honest and say that if I can cook, *anyone* can! Let me give you an example. A couple of years ago some good friends of ours invited us to spend Easter with them at their gorgeous farm in Sydney's Southern Highlands. It gets pretty cold down there in the autumn, so on a chilly Sunday morning I decided to get up early and cook porridge for everyone.

One of the other guests there that weekend was my friend's mother, the renowned chef Suzanne Gibbs, herself the daughter of Australia's most celebrated cook, Margaret Fulton.

Thinking I had done a pretty good job of the porridge, I was looking forward to receiving some complimentary feedback when I noticed Suzanne peering into the saucepan on the stove.

'Is this supposed to be porridge?' she queried with a smile.

Her husband, Rob, who had been tucking into his bowl, looked up questioningly.

'No, Suzanne. It's Bircher muesli,' he replied. 'At least I think it is.'

Some people would be mortified by having a famous chef unable to recognise their preparation of such a simple dish, but I took it in my stride (with the help of extensive therapy!). After all, I knew that I'd had many more successes than failures. It's like anything in life: the more you do it, the better you get. And the quicker you get at it, too.

The major factor in our country's burgeoning waistlines, and the accompanying decline in our nation's health, is the lack of confidence in the kitchen and the negative headspace we have when it comes to cooking. And I'm talking about real cooking. Not taking some chicken nuggets out of the freezer and sticking them

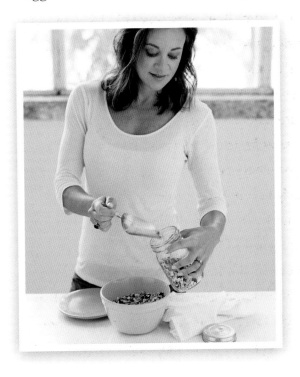

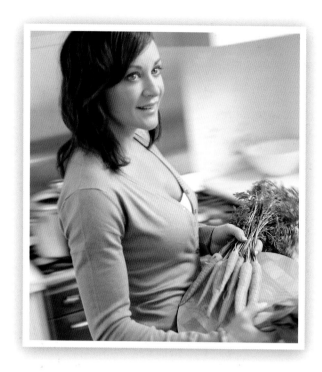

in the oven for ten minutes. I'm talking about taking a piece of fresh chicken, scattering it with herbs and chilli and putting it in the steamer for ten minutes. The cost and preparation time are about the same. The similarity ends when you taste them – one has all the flavour of the cardboard box it came in, and the other one melts in your mouth and tastes, well, like chicken!

I hear a lot of people tell me that they think it's all too hard. 'Who can be bothered?' they say, which is pretty understandable when we've convinced ourselves that takeaway is quicker, cheaper, and even at times healthier than cooking at home. This couldn't be further from the truth.

People selling food want it to taste good to keep you coming back, and they don't think twice about adding ingredients that will make their dishes oily, salty, sweet or fatty. By the time you've waited for takeaway or home delivery you could easily have made something nutritious *and* eaten it. And as for the dollars and cents, I've done the numbers and it really is cheaper to eat at home than to eat out – especially when you factor in the cost of petrol, the alcoholic drinks you'll probably buy and that you won't get any leftovers for lunch or another meal.

We're so busy doing other things – working, socialising, following hobbies and interests – that we've allowed food companies to take responsibility for what we eat. And that's where it goes wrong. *As soon as you let someone else be in charge of what you eat you're in trouble!*

Once upon a time we would only ever eat what we grew in our own gardens or bought from the local market. It would be seasonal and fresh. Our choices were governed by where we lived, the time of year, and what was readily available. Sure, we had to preserve like mad every year so that we could have summer fruits in winter, but for the most part, that was it.

Nowadays, we have an overwhelming abundance of choice, much of which we don't actually need, all driven by the overpowering volume of advertising that smothers us every day. It's got to the point where many people just don't know what good, simple, healthy eating is any more. You wouldn't believe how many of my clients say, 'Just tell me what to eat!'

So here they are: the recipes you need to help

you lose weight. In Part 3, I give you 100 tried-and-true recipes, including *all* of my favourites, and every one of them is low in calories and high in flavour. Because I'm incredibly busy, and I know you are too, my recipes are always simple to prepare and easy to follow. Please don't be overwhelmed by how many there are – I just wanted to give you lots and lots of choices. Once you have mastered two or three of them, you'll feel your confidence blossom, and you'll be bursting to try the others. Also, I encourage you to experiment: get a few recipes under your belt, change a couple of key ingredients and 'voila!' you have yourself a new meal!

But of course, knowing *what* to cook is only part of the story, you also need to know *how* to set yourself up for successful weight management, and in Part 1 I give you practical tips on counting calories and getting organised in the kitchen. In Part 2 I've designed a 12-Week Menu Plan, plus there are detox and exercise tips to get you started on your journey to a leaner, healthier you.

I have written this book to show you how much easier, how much cheaper and how much quicker it is to prepare your own meals. Confidence in the kitchen is the key to weight management, so I'm giving you recipes that will help you not only lose the kilos that you want to lose, but also *maintain* control of your weight. In doing so you'll regain your health, vitality and energy. But do you know what the

best thing will be? You will lose weight by eating *really good food*. And believe me, by following these recipes you will learn to love good food – *really* love it. You will feel excited about cooking healthy food rather than be scared of it or think of it as the enemy.

Be ready, though. Once you begin to eat the delicious, fresh wholefoods in my recipes and understand more about food and nutrition, junk food will never look or taste the same.

One of the most amazing transformations I see in my work with *The Biggest Loser* contestants is their attitude to food. Many of the contestants at the beginning of the show don't have a clue about how to prepare a meal: for some, 'cooking' means putting frozen pies in the oven. There is also plenty of confusion about what constitutes 'healthy' food, plus lots of turned-up noses to fresh vegetables. By the end of the show they are cooking up a storm in the kitchen, have an informed grasp of nutrition, and love the taste of fresh wholefood. They tell me that their tastebuds have changed and that they've not only lost the desire to eat salty, fatty, processed foods, but also feel bloated and sluggish when they do.

You are about to take charge of your kitchen, and in the process take charge of your weight and your life. You are about to take back control. What you learn will last you a lifetime and will be passed on to your own children. How exciting is that?

Let's get cooking!

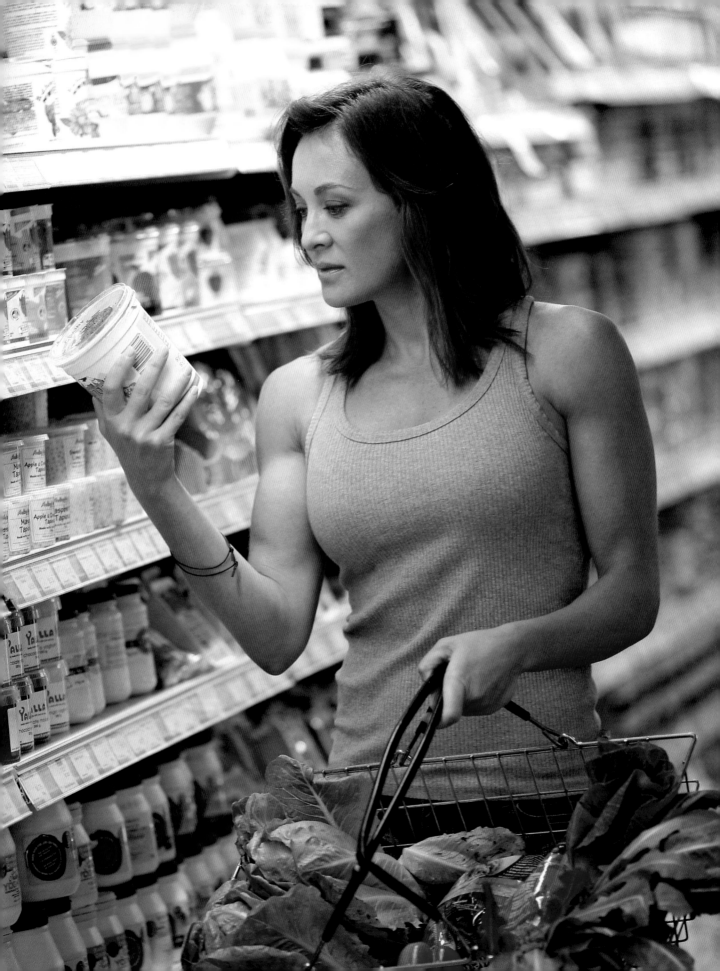

Part 1

The rules

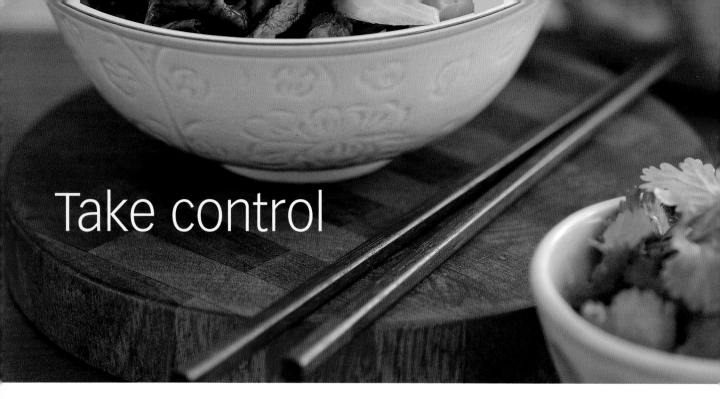

Take control

In this section I want to explain how the food you eat contributes to your weight and overall health, and how you can take control of what you eat by getting organised in your kitchen.

Change your habits

If you are tired and lethargic and feel like a zombie extra from *Return of the Living Dead* I guarantee that you are not feeding yourself properly. That's what I'm here for – to show you simple, nutritious recipes that will give you energy *and* help you lose weight. You see, it's no coincidence that highly nutritious food is also low in calories, so as well as helping you out with your time management and fatigue, I'm going to strip a couple of kilos off you on the way! Yep, it's your lucky day!

Now it's all very well to have a hundred easy recipes, but how can you be sure that you will control your portions? That you won't reach for the biscuits/cakes/chocolates as a reward for eating such a healthy meal? How do you change the old thought patterns and break the old habits that have been keeping you stuck in a body that you are not particularly proud of?

We are all creatures of habit. Over the years I've come to recognise some of the most common habits that lead to weight problems, and I'm guilty of doing some of them myself!

- Having a biscuit/muffin/cake every time we have a cup of tea.
- Reaching for the chocolate/wine/biscuits whenever we feel overwhelmed/depressed/celebratory.
- Going back for seconds even though we feel full.

- Skipping meals and then stuffing ourselves later on.
- Mindlessly eating in front of the TV.

Even though these habits don't sound too dramatic on their own, when you add them together, and repeat them daily for a few months or even years, the result can be disastrous. But the great news is that habits are learned, so they can be unlearned – they can

be *replaced*. It's time for you to come up with a game plan for what you will do *from this point forward* when you've had a bad day, broken up with a partner, had a fight with your mum, got a pay rise, are celebrating a birthday or are just plain bored. Do something which you *know* will

Anthony's secret

I worked with a male client a few years back whose story has never left me. Although he exercised regularly he was quite overweight. He even had a personal trainer for about a year. His problem was binge eating. When he was in the company of family and friends he ate very little and always chose super-healthy foods, but when he was home alone he would go crazy, particularly at night.

Eventually, after I asked many, many questions, he confided in me that he would never eat a lot in front of people because he felt that they would judge him. For the first time he had shared with someone the behaviour patterns that had resulted in his weight issues, but his honesty with me was in fact the turning point for him to begin working through it.

Hiding food in wardrobes as a child, lolly wrappers under the bed, eating in the car, pretending to be buying food for other people, offering to go out to buy coffee for work mates so he could buy muffins and eat them before he got back to the office, eating in the stairwell at work, eating two dinners – one at home and one out –

the list was disturbing and endless.

As we worked together, over time it became apparent that this was only part of the story. Yes, he felt people watching him eat were judging him, but there was more to it than that. By not eating in front of others he was able to deny his problem. Although he was embarrassed by his actions, no-one else knew about them so there was no need for him to *do* anything about them. Because he was putting so much energy into hiding his eating, he was actually giving it an enormous amount of attention. The more he tried to hide it, the bigger the issue became.

He told me that most of his family and friends truly believed that his being overweight was a result of genetics – that he was one of those people who just can't lose weight. He was living a lie and it was impacting not only on his physical health, but also his mental and spiritual health.

The breakthrough came when he was able to admit, out loud, that he was actually lying, to his friends, family and work colleagues, but most significantly to himself. The relief he felt was incredible. He felt energised and alive and ready to take on the world.

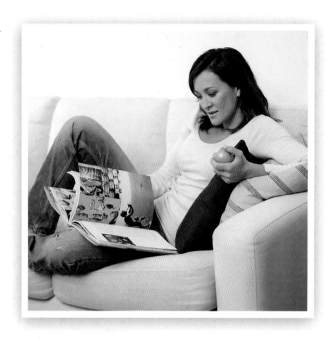

make you feel better. Exchange your *bad* habit for a *good* habit – something that will make you smile rather than feel ashamed when you wake up the next morning.

Good habits

- Eating breakfast every day.
- Spending the first half hour of every day exercising.
- Eating a piece of fruit for dessert, but only doing this twice a week.
- Brushing your teeth immediately after dinner, then having no more food.

Bad habits

- **Eating takeaway/out all the time**. Remember – your kitchen is ground control for weight management. Chefs are experts at making food extra tasty by using lots of butter, salt, sugar and oils.

- **Finishing off the kids' dinners**. Put them in a container for lunch tomorrow. Think of the money you'll save!

- **Drinking alcohol**. Apart from being 'empty' calories (in other words although it's a carbohydrate, it's technically not a food because it has no nutritional value), you'll get smashed and make dumb food choices. Don't let a few wines ruin all that clean eating and hard training!

- **Eating anywhere but at the dinner table**. If you eat while driving, walking, watching TV, standing in front of the fridge or pantry, it's harder for you to stay in control. When you eat on the couch, you associate sitting on the couch with eating. So every time you sit on the couch, usually in front of a television, you find yourself reaching for food and you *don't acknowledge what you are eating*. It's no coincidence that many obese families don't have a dining table – they always eat on the couch. By sitting down at a table, without distractions, you can enjoy your meal and really taste it.

- **Going back for seconds.** This is a major no-no. You don't need the extra food – it's just that your body is used to huge portions. It's time to train it to have smaller serves.

- **Eating while you cook.** Another bad habit for obvious reasons. Don't drink alcohol while you cook, either – it only makes it harder to make good decisions, such as *not* eating while you're cooking.

Count your calories

If you are in the market to drop some weight, whether it's the last 5 kilograms (always the toughest!) or 20 to 40 of the little suckers, you will be *treading water* if you don't understand some basic principles about the food you are eating – namely, the amount of energy (calories/kilojoules) it contains.

Put simply, to lose weight you have to be taking in *fewer calories* ('energy in') than you are burning up ('energy out') to put you into a calorie deficit. I am yet to work with a client for whom the energy in/energy out principle doesn't work. Sometimes prescription drugs and hormonal imbalances can make it tougher to shift weight, but even when clients have these issues, I've still had success using the right nutrition and exercise.

Now you may notice I prefer to use calories, but that's because my heart-rate monitor counts calories and all the fitness equipment in health clubs does too. Feel free, though, to use kilojoules if you prefer: 1 calorie equals 4.2 kilojoules, so simply multiply your calories by 4.2 to get kilojoules, or divide your kilojoules by 4.2 to get calories.

When I work with my clients I try to keep it as simple as possible. Depending on your age, exercise levels and incidental activity throughout the day, the following is a good guide to the number of calories you should be taking on board:

Recommended calories per day

Girls 1200–1500 calories	3 meals each at around 300–350 calories plus 1 or 2 snacks at around 100–150 calories
Guys 1300–1800 calories	3 meals each at around 400–450 calories plus 1 or 2 snacks at around 200 calories

Adding up your daily calorie intake not only teaches you to identify calorie-dense foods, but also makes you feel that *you* are in control of your weight and your life. I'm not suggesting that you must do this forever, or become socially unacceptable by adding up loudly at a dinner party, but it's the best way to get your hands back on the steering wheel.

To help you with calorie control, I have designed all the breakfast, lunch and dinner recipes so that you will only be taking in around 300 to 400 calories per serve. If you are used to eating much larger portions of heavier, calorie-dense food, my 12-Week Menu Plan will result in some dramatic weight loss, even if you don't do *any* training. I know a 100 kilogram non-exercising male who was able to drop 10 kilograms over three weeks simply by cutting out all junk food, beer and soft drink! Impressive! And even if you already consider yourself to be a reasonably healthy eater and regular exerciser but have a few kilos to lose, you can expect to drop between 1 and 3 per cent of your body weight each week by following my menu plan. This is because the calories are tight, and twelve weeks is sufficient time to develop the eating habits that will last you a lifetime.

If you are in the market for some *fast* results you will need to combine healthy eating with training to bump up the calories you are burning. My book *Crunch Time* has a 12-week workout program that will see you dropping some major kilos. (Just so you know, to lose 1 kilogram in a week, you need to have a deficit of around 7500 calories.)

Control your portions

Exercise aside, most people are overweight because they *eat too much*; they are taking in way more fuel than their bodies actually need. They're used to eating huge serves of meat or sugary carbs and having their vegies or salad as a garnish (if at all).

One way to help with portion control is to divide up the plate. *Three quarters* of your plate should be covered with salad or vegetables. Half of that should be predominantly green leafy vegies, and the remainder should be low-GI vegetables such as sweet potato or cauliflower, or some cold beans in the summer. The other *quarter* should be protein such as fish, chicken breast or lean red meat.

Most vegetables are very low in calories, so it's not too hard to work out portion sizes. The following is a *very rough* guide that I use when I'm shopping or preparing food:

100 g of salad vegies (lettuce, tomatoes, capsicum, bok choy, cabbage, zucchini, eggplant)	**20 calories**
100 g of 'light' vegetables (carrots, onions, swede, turnip, leeks)	**25 calories**
100 g of 'heavy' vegetables (sweet potato, pumpkin, parsnip)	**50 calories**

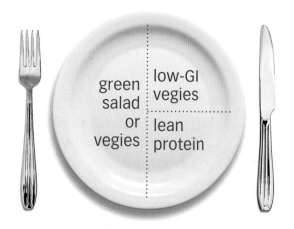

The calorie content for meat and fish varies, so portion sizes need to be adjusted. White fish, seafood and kangaroo have the lowest number of calories, followed by chicken, salmon and red meat. Here is a rough guide that I use when I'm shopping or preparing a meal:

1 g of white fish, seafood, kangaroo	1 calorie
1 g of chicken, tuna	1.5 calories
1 g of red meat, salmon	2 calories

TIP – Every now and then go back and measure or weigh your food again just to keep you on track. It can be easy to get heavy-handed over time.

Diana, the queen of denial

I met Diana a couple of years back in a Sydney gym. I don't usually get tears from my clients until we're halfway through the first training session, but on this occasion I managed to excel myself and Diana was crying in the first two minutes of our initial conversation.

Diana was quite overweight, and explained that she'd put the weight on with her first baby, and that it had stayed. In fact, it had compounded. Her words were: 'I desperately want to lose the weight, I hate it.'

She was at the gym, which I thought was a good start, but obviously, she was struggling. She was telling me all the stuff that she thought I wanted to hear like: 'I come to the gym three times a week, and I actually eat very healthy food.'

Experience told me that Diana wasn't trying to convince me, but was trying to convince herself. I knew that if she was telling herself she was trying hard to eat well and exercise, then her weight problem 'wasn't her fault'. It gave her permission to be a victim, and in doing so, allowed her to perpetuate her unhealthy lifestyle. So, I cut to the chase.

'Okay. Tell me what you had for dinner last night.'

'Oh, um, spaghetti bolognese – that's my kids' favourite.'

'Right. So what was your serving size and did you go back for seconds?' I asked.

Bang. Her face told me everything. Her serving size was the same as her husband's – large. And, yes, she not only went back for seconds but finished off the kids' meals, because, hey, you can't waste food right? Then gradually it came out that she'd also had some garlic bread, half a bottle of wine and a little Easter egg or five after dinner.

'But that's not a normal night's dinner!' she claimed.

I wasn't sold. 'You say you want to lose the weight desperately but you are knowingly sabotaging your efforts. You say you know what you need to do to get there, and yet you're not doing it. *You deserve to have whatever it is that you desire.* If you desire to get fit, feel healthy, feel sexy and lose some weight, then do it girlfriend! Stop talking about it and playing the victim and get on with it!

'Keep coming to the gym but start looking after your nutrition as well. Otherwise you're getting nowhere. You deserve more than this.'

There were tears. It's not easy having straight conversations, but she knew and I knew that she had been denying what was actually going on.

It took a little while after our conversation for the penny to drop, but she told me later she had still been in the headspace of 'being on a diet'. She had not fully embraced a good diet and exercise as her new way of life.

'Once I realised that this is how I *choose* to live, this is just how I am all the time, it all clicked into place. Yeah, every now and again I will have a splurge, but most of the time I don't even like it because of how it makes me feel afterwards. I have way more energy and vitality when I am eating fresh food. Plus, I look back on how I used to eat and *I was kidding* myself that I ate healthily. I really didn't, and everything was in massive portions.'

I continued to see Diana at the gym over the next year, and she completely transformed herself. She looked amazing and dropped quite a few sizes. Good on her for doing the hard work and addressing what was really going on. She had stopped the rollercoaster, stepped off and walked away. Very cool.

Bear in mind that these are rough guides only, and the calorie content will vary depending on how it's cooked. It's not an exact science, but it's handy if you don't want to consult a calorie counter every time you're in the supermarket.

The next step is to learn what portion sizes look like. I have all my clients invest in a set of kitchen scales as it's really the only way to know. Once you have weighed your food a couple of times you'll quickly get to know what 100 g of red meat looks like, or 200 g of white fish so you won't have to do it all the time.

The same applies to measuring. For example, measure out half a cup of rolled oats or muesli and get to know what it looks like in your bowl. After a while you won't need to do much weighing or measuring and when you eat out you'll have a good idea of how much is on your plate.

Eat regularly

The number one bad habit for *all* of my overweight clients, without exception, is that they *don't eat breakfast*. They also barely eat lunch or only have a high-carb snack such as a muffin. Then, having starved themselves, they gorge themselves crazy from the moment they walk through the door in the evening till they go to bed.

Now this sounds like a lesson from the school of the bleeding obvious, but the best time to eat is *when we need the energy*, and for most of us that will be in the morning and at lunchtime, depending on our incidental

activity and whether we are exercising in the morning or the afternoon. This is why your breakfast is *so* important – a nutritious, low-GI carbohydrate early meal sets us up for a successful day. It also ensures that we don't feel hungry midmorning and reach for that sugary, processed snack.

Following my 12-Week Menu Plan means you will now be feeding yourself well during the day and won't *need* a monster dinner when you are winding down at the end of the day. Dinners will be a bit smaller than you are used to. But don't stress! My dinner recipes taste amazing and are purposely designed to work for all family members, whether they need to lose weight or not. Plus, you'll sleep better when you don't have such a full stomach.

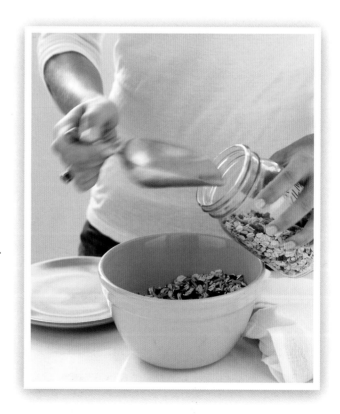

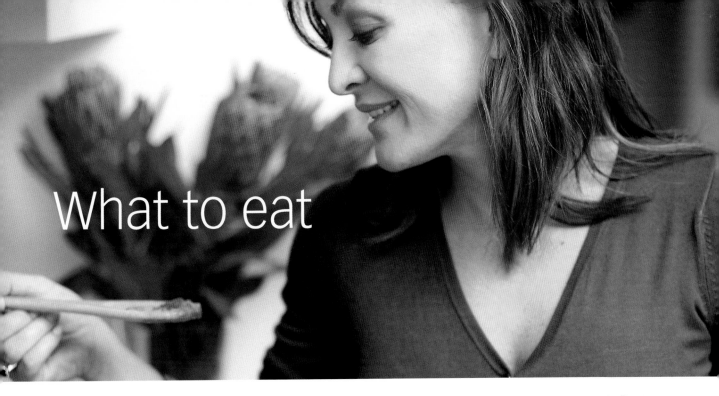

What to eat

I eat wholefoods – that means food that has been refined as little as possible, if at all. Wholefoods include unprocessed meat, poultry, fish, fruit, vegetables, nuts and grains and are what we call 'nutrient-dense' foods. These foods usually contain fewer calories, so we can eat more of them, though there are some exceptions – a large avocado, for example, is a whopping 500 calories, and cashew nuts are 10 calories each. In general, most of your food needs to look as close to its natural state as possible and be fresh and seasonal.

Vegetables and fruit

Vegetables are jam-packed with vitamins, minerals, antioxidants and other nutrients. Eat them cooked or raw and in as many different colours as possible – especially green ones.

Fresh is absolutely best, but you can use frozen or tinned occasionally for convenience – just be wary of additives and sugar. Because vegetables are so low in calories they are pretty much open slather when it comes to your daily intake – you can usually eat as much as you want without breaking your calorie limit.

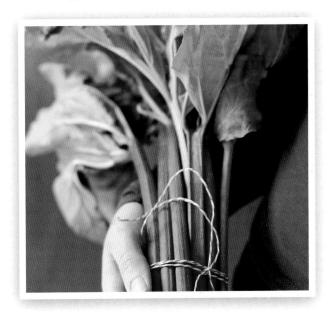

You'll notice that all my recipes feature vegetables and/or fruit and that the proportion of vegies is always larger than the meat. Vegies are the rock star attraction – the meat is just the back-up singer.

Fruit is also unbeatable when it comes to good health and I always have a full fruit bowl in my kitchen. Again, fresh is best when it comes to taste, so buy seasonal. Fruits are higher in energy than vegetables, which is why they are so fantastic for breakfast or for a morning snack. Only have two pieces a day, though, as the calories can mount up.

I steer clear of fruit juices as they are usually full of sugar and contain no fibre. I'd rather have the piece of fruit itself and get all the fibre as well. If I do have a freshly squeezed juice it will always be a vegie juice rather than a fruit juice. A small-sized carrot, ginger and mint is my fave.

Protein

Protein is essential for the building and repair of all body tissue and is found in meat, fish and shellfish, dairy products, seeds, nuts, and legumes (lentils and beans). For dinner, I try to stick to only two red-meat dishes a week (one of which is usually kangaroo), two chicken meals, one fish and two vegetarian dishes. For lunch I rarely have red meat, mostly sticking to vegetables or chicken, and occasionally fish.

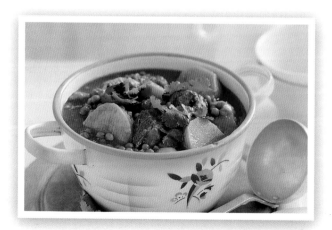

Kangaroo

This is at the top of my list of lean meats. It's high in protein, low in fat (less than 2 per cent) and high in omega 3 which assists in lowering cholesterol. It's also *super* low in calories – even lower than a lot of fish! It's also organic (no hormones or chemicals) and is more environmentally friendly than other sources of red meat as kangaroos produce no methane gas, and being soft-footed create no soil degradation. They are virtually drought proof and require far less food than cattle. They spend their entire lives in their natural habitat, and are humanely culled by experts.

You will find four fabulous recipes for kangaroo in this book (see pages 106–9 and 183–5) and most of the beef recipes can be adapted for kangaroo.

Beef and other red meat

When it comes to other red meats, organic is great but can be quite expensive. When buying beef, I only buy grass-fed, never grain-fed because the meat is significantly lower in nutrients and higher in fat. Plus, these poor animals are kept in feedlots whereas their grass-fed counterparts live on open pasture closer to their natural state.

Buy what you can afford and know where the meat has come from by reading the label or asking your butcher. Keep in mind though that I am asking you to eat less meat than you may have in the past, so you may be able to afford better quality cuts. Remember to always go for the lean cuts and to trim off any fat.

Fats

Fats are found in vegetable oils, meat, fish, nuts and dairy products (milk, butter, cream, cheese, yoghurt). They are an important energy source and essential for certain body functions, but are *very* high in calories, which is why I eat only very small amounts of them. There are also good fats (mono- and poly-unsaturated) and bad fats (hydrogenated and saturated), and we have to be careful to eat the right kinds, and not too much of them, because the truth is your butt doesn't know the difference between a good fat and a bad fat!

To get my quota of fats (they should make up 20–30 per cent of our daily calorie intake), I eat plenty of fish, a few eggs, use a little olive oil in my cooking and occasionally have:

- Low-fat cottage cheese on carrot and celery sticks
- Low-fat cottage cheese on a piece of toast
- Some full-flavoured parmesan cheese grated over a salad
- A small tub of diet yoghurt
- A dollop of full-fat Greek-style yoghurt on breakfast fruit
- Low-fat high-calcium milk in tea or on oats.

What does low-GI mean?

Carbohydrates are actually found in most foods (including vegetables, nuts, seeds, fruit and milk), so limiting grain-based foods (bread, rice, cereals, pasta) means we still get plenty of energy from our fruit and vegetables.

The best carbohydrates are the ones that are absorbed slowly into our bloodstream because this keeps our blood sugar levels more stable, and helps us to feel fuller for longer. These are the carbs with a low glycaemic index (GI) of less than 55. High-GI carbs have an index of more than 70, and intermediate carbs are those in between. High GI is not necessarily a bad thing, especially the night before a race or a mean training session, but if you want to lose weight, you need to stick to low-GI foods.

Low-GI fruit and vegetables include apples, bananas, cherries, grapefruit, grapes, kiwi fruit, legumes, oranges, peaches, pears, peas, plums, strawberries, sweet potatoes and sweetcorn.

But GI is only half the story – we also have to consider **glycaemic load**, which takes into account the size of the portion that's being eaten. A slice of watermelon, for example, is high GI (72), but its glycaemic load is just 4. This is because although the sugar gets into your system quickly, there simply isn't enough of it in a 120 g slice to significantly elevate your blood sugar levels. A bar of chocolate, on the other hand, is low GI (49), but its glycaemic load is 15. Glycaemic loads are low if less than 10, moderate up to 19 and high at 20 or more.

Fish and seafood

I love fish and seafood. It's generally only around 1 calorie per gram and is really versatile as you'll see from my fabulous recipes. I seldom eat battered fish (maybe once on a summer holiday sitting on the beach) because deep frying *doubles* the calories. Plus it's often deep fried in trans-fats (which have been linked to cancer), and because I really don't know what's in the batter, or underneath it for that matter, it breaks one of my golden rules – *always know exactly what you're eating.*

TIP – Be <u>very</u> careful with cheese, as it can blow your calorie quota in a flash!

Dairy products

Some of us have a total aversion to dairy products for various reasons, but I like to use them a little in my diet. When it comes to dairy products, you need to be aware that 'low fat' *isn't* necessarily 'low calorie'. That's because the fat content is what makes dairy food tasty, and once manufacturers take it out, they'll often replace it with sugar so that people will still like the taste.

The bottom line with dairy is that you need to make a little go a long way. Some of the low-fat, low-calorie cheeses can have very little taste and you can wind up eating more than you realise. I prefer to have a full-flavoured cheese that I can actually taste and enjoy, but only have a very small portion. As always, it's about reading the label, knowing the calories and nailing your portion sizes.

Wholegrain foods

Wholegrain foods are simply those that use the entire grain. The dark outside layer contains a lot of important nutrients, and in most grains it is rich in fibre. Refined white flour (used in most breads, biscuits, cereals, etc.) has had this outer layer removed, so is far less nutritious, and is virtually useless when it comes to keeping us 'regular'. Yet we are so used to filling up on these refined carbohydrates that many of us have never even tried wholegrain alternatives.

Bread

Make sure you always buy wholegrain or wholemeal flat bread, loaves or rolls – it's more nutritious. I don't eat a lot of bread, and when I do it's always in the morning or for lunch, never at night, and it's always soy and linseed or a good-quality wholegrain. When using rolls, scoop out the inside so you can put in more filling.

Rice

Rice is an excellent way of pumping up the calorie count of a stir-fry for growing kids or any manual workers in the household. For weight-loss candidates though, rice should generally be avoided. Brown rice has a lower GI than white. The best white rice choices are doongara and basmati as they are low GI. I occasionally eat these for lunch, but rarely eat them at night.

Pasta

Pasta often gets a bum rap, even though it's an excellent source of energy. As with rice and bread, portion size is critical, followed by what you put on it, and then the time of day you eat it. I reserve my pasta dishes for lunches, and in small portions, and always follow them with a smashing training session later on. You'll notice in the spaghetti bolognese recipe (page 170) that I substitute greens for pasta, though you can serve wholemeal pasta to growing children or anyone who needs the extra calories.

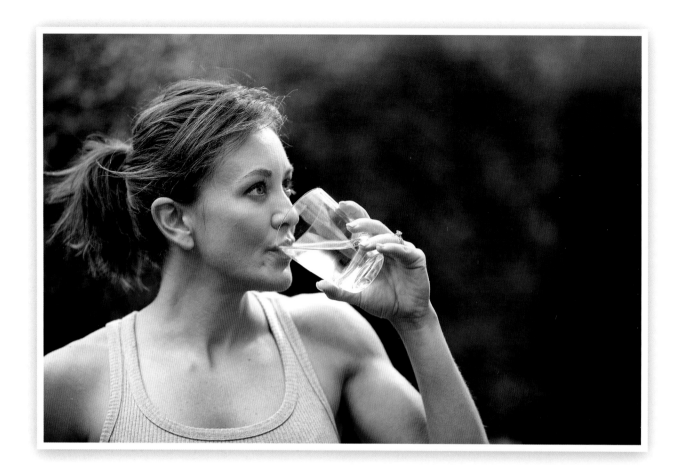

Noodles

Noodles are usually made from wheat or rice flour, and soak up the flavours of the foods that they are served with. Portions need to be small – half to three-quarters of a cup (cooked). Avoid instant noodles as they can be loaded with salt and have a higher GI than their fresh counterparts.

Lentils, beans and other legumes

Legumes are often seen as food for vegetarians, or are criticised for being a bit long-winded (pardon the pun) to prepare, but I'm here to tell you that they are a *super food*, particularly lentils, which are dead easy to cook and highly nutritious.

They have some unique advantages over other foods – they are cheap (and I mean *cheap*!), they last just about forever and they are really versatile in the kitchen. They are packed with protein and low-GI carbohydrates along with cholesterol lowering fibre, B group vitamins and folate. I actually use them instead of minced beef in my yummy lentil shepherd's pie (see page 115).

Water

Water is needed for most bodily functions – digestion, the transportation of nutrients, the removal of waste and toxins, cushioning of tissues, organs and joints, regulating temperature, maintaining good skin and more.

We need at least six glasses (1.5 litres) of water a day in order to maintain a healthy body, more if we are training. Like the majority of us, I have to admit I don't always drink enough water, particularly during winter. However, when I do, I notice that my skin is not as dry, nor is my scalp, and the extra trip or two to the bathroom could be considered 'incidental exercise' thus helping me burn up calories!

Interestingly, a lot of the times that I think I'm hungry I'm actually thirsty, and once I have a glass of water, I'm no longer tempted to have an extra snack. I aim to drink between 2 and 3 litres of water a day.

> TIP – Use a water bottle that you fill up from home. We don't need any more plastic bottles.

If you're struggling to drink your six glasses per day, try a squeeze of lemon or lime juice in your water, or drink sparkling mineral water. Having a bottle of water on your desk, in your car or in your handbag increases the likelihood of reaching your daily target. Sometimes I drink it from a wine glass to make it feel a bit more special! Whatever! Up the water levels and feel the difference.

Desserts and treats?

My clients who are serious about losing weight *never* eat dessert. End of story. I can hear a lot of my colleagues saying 'As soon as you tell someone they can't have something they will want it' or 'You should allow them to have it when they feel they can handle it.' But to them I say phooey! If I have an adult in my charge who seriously wants to lose weight, take back control and responsibility, then I will insist that they steer clear of the food which has obviously held them back.

I work with many people who need to break old habits and patterns, particularly when it comes to sweet food at night, and having no dessert is a useful drill. Why? Because the satisfaction you feel when you are able to say 'no' to a food that you used to buckle at the sight of is powerful. You are in control instead of the other way around.

So why do I have desserts in my book? Well, the answer is that I *do* allow my clients to have a weekly treat meal once we've been working together for a few weeks and my clients have had some great results. (Funnily enough, most of them choose not to!) Also, if you are at your goal weight a small, low-calorie dessert once in a while isn't going to break the bank. I guess it all comes down to how quickly you want to reach your goal. Just know, though, that no dessert will *ever* leave you feeling as good as you will when you fit into your old jeans!

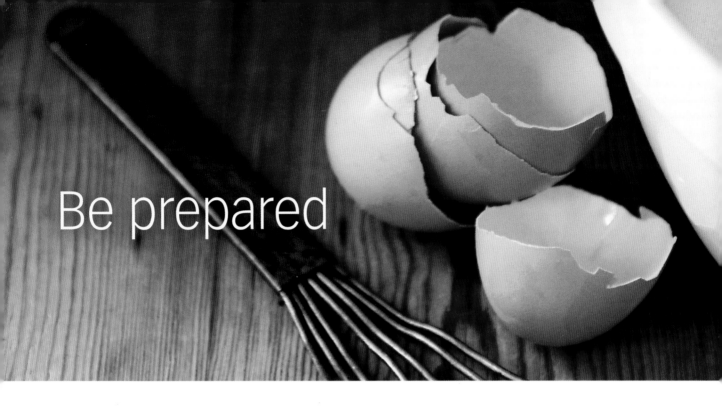

Be prepared

Being organised is probably the single most important element of good nutrition – seriously! So always have your ingredients fresh/defrosted and ready to go. Keep a shopping list on the go (the menu plan in Part 2 will help with this) and always be sure to restock your fridge, freezer and pantry with the ingredients you need for your week's meals.

This may sound over the top if you are used to 'making it up as you go along', but believe me, being disorganised is the reason so many people fall back into old habits (i.e. takeaway, frozen dinners). If you are serious about managing your weight you have to be prepared to put some time in the kitchen.

I love a meal which can almost 'cook itself' while I jump in the shower so that when I come out it's just about done. Defrosting and reheating a dish I made on the weekend is the easiest option, but I have dozens of quick and easy dishes in my tool kit, and I share them all with you in Part 3.

It all comes down to being prepared.

When I know I'll be coming home at around eight o'clock in the evening cold and hungry, that morning I might take a piece of fish out of the freezer (that I bought fresh on the weekend) and pop it into the fridge so that it will defrost throughout the day. That night, as soon as I walk in, I'll turn on the oven, put the fish in an aluminium foil 'boat', chop up some shallots, garlic, chilli and ginger and scatter them on top, squeeze in a full lemon and add some lemon zest (that's grated rind for us non-chefs). Then the fish goes in the oven while I have my shower.

As soon as I get out I pop some green vegies into the steamer for a few minutes and my dinner is pretty much ready to serve. It's light on calories, big on taste, easy on the wallet and quick to prepare – around fifteen minutes tops, plus I'm showered and in my PJs!

You can be this efficient too – you only need to be *prepared*, to know at the start of the day what you're going to be making that night for dinner and have the ingredients ready. If you don't have the ingredients in the house, don't worry – you can still grab them on the way home, but what you *don't* want to do is end up staring into an empty fridge saying 'What am I going to eat tonight? Might have to dial a pizza . . .'

It's also about looking ahead and knowing what you're going to eat tomorrow and the coming weekend. 'Will there be decent food at the football on Saturday? Or should I pack some salad sandwiches?' When you are organised you are *back in control*. You aren't letting others be responsible for what you eat. When you let go of that responsibility, when you let others determine how your body is nourished, you lose control of your weight.

Super-efficient cooking

Part of being organised is being more efficient in the way you prepare meals. Each time I cook, I try to make more than one meal. By doubling the quantities, for example, I can cook two meals, one to be eaten right away and the other frozen or refrigerated for later (see my spicy beef and vegetable meatloaf, page 174). In the 12-Week Menu Plan in Part 2, you'll find that many of the weekend meals are designed especially to be used for weekday lunches later in the week.

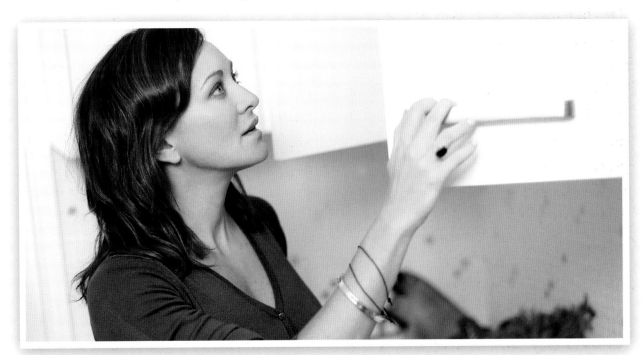

I often cook up extra ingredients to use as the basis for another meal, too. For example, sometimes I partly steam extra vegetables so that I can bake them the next night with some fish (and they'll take the same amount of time to cook), or I poach an extra breast of chicken (see Chinese poached chicken, page 161) to be used for sandwiches or wraps for lunch the next day. I also use the liquid from my poached chicken as a stock for other dishes, such as soup.

Now soup would have to be the best example of an efficient meal. For my chicken and vegetable soup with silverbeet (page 74), I often make up more of the vegetable stock base, and then reheat this adding some beef or chicken to make a delicious meal. Or I may ladle the soup base into a bowl and then pop a handful of English spinach or sliced bok choy on top and simply let the heat of the soup wilt the greens. It gives the soup a nice fresh feel even though it's been reheated.

Right now you're probably thinking 'Eeeghh! It all sounds too hard!' But you have to trust me on this. Once you get started it is surprisingly easy and very rewarding. And if I can do this, I'm telling you, anyone can!

My favourite methods

I prefer cooking methods like steaming, stir-frying and grilling because they are so much quicker and I know I'll be able to savour the taste of every vegetable, herb and spice. Boiling is not my style as it can zap out all the flavour, and frying or deep-frying food in loads of oil simply adds way too many calories.

Stir-frying

Stir-fries feature lots of vegetables and so fit my profile of being nutritious, easy and delicious. You require barely any oil, just a light spray. Smothering your stir-fry with sauces (soy, hoisin, oyster, etc.) will also blow out the calories so watch the portions. I prefer to use fresh herbs for extra flavour. Also, watch your

Clean up your pantry

Before you get cooking, you'll need to clean up your pantry. It's time to say goodbye to some old friends who are now your enemies – you know who I mean: the chips, lollies and chocolates, the sweet biscuits and cakes, the frozen dinners and packet mixes, the soft drinks, the cheesy, salty crap-in-a-box. The rest of your family might have something to say about this, however, this is about *your* health. *You* are the adult. You are the one who's paying the bills. And you are the one who is responsible for your children's health.

By the way, my view on parents who regularly give their children junk food to reward them or to pacify them is very clear-cut. I see them as engaging in a form of child abuse.

As parents, it is your responsibility to teach your children good eating habits, because these habits will last a lifetime. Do you want your children to develop the bad habits you are working so hard to change? Be the one to break the cycle.

cooking times. The vegies should still have a little crunch to them and be bright in colour.

I'm a big fan of olive oil spray. A three-second spray is enough to coat a wok (or a baking dish) and is only about 10–15 calories. You can also buy refillable spray pumps, which work out even cheaper. I use only high-quality cold-pressed virgin olive oil, which tastes better. (I don't use very much so I want to be able to taste it!) And don't get caught thinking that 'light' olive oils have less calories than ordinary olive oils – the 'light' refers to the flavour. The calories are exactly the same.

The other reason stir-fries are so brilliant is that they are so versatile. Once you master them you can always change a few key ingredients and have a whole new meal without having to learn how to cook a whole new recipe! It's a win–win. I believe that this is the secret to becoming a better cook – experimenting. Some of my best meals have turned up purely by chance because I could only use what I had in the fridge and the pantry at the time.

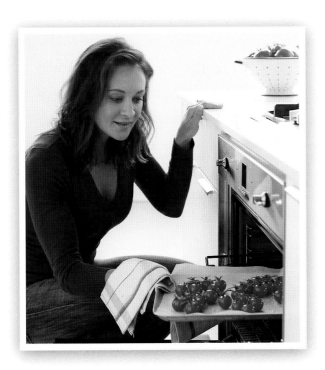

Steaming

We steam *a lot* in our house. It's the healthiest way to prepare vegetables, and is also a great way to cook chicken or fish. Get yourself set up with a good steaming saucepan that can take plenty of vegies. The ones with separate inserts are handy as you can steam a variety of foods on one stove element or burner, saving time and gas/electricity. Try popping in a sprig of rosemary, clove of garlic or a bay leaf with your vegies to give them a fabulous aromatic flavour. It also makes the kitchen smell great!

Grilling and char-grilling

Grilling on the barbecue is another healthy way to cook and is super easy too, but don't overdo the oil, otherwise your healthy meal can quickly degenerate into a calorie-fest. One of my favourite dishes is barbecued vegetables: eggplant, mushrooms, onions, thinly sliced zucchini – yum! So don't think it's all snags and steaks.

Try using a ridged, non-stick char-grill pan on your stovetop. They are a really clever way to cook as the ridges help to drain away any excess fat if you're cooking meat and therefore keep the calories down. I use mine all the time and you'll see it in many of my recipes.

Poaching

I can't tell you how many times I used to cook a chicken breast only to find it was dry and stringy. Welcome to the wonderful world of poaching! It is *so* simple to poach chicken that you'll be kicking yourself that you didn't discover this *fantastic* cooking method earlier.

The great thing is that you can add herbs and other flavours to the poaching water to make it taste delicious. *Plus* you can keep the water for stock. Check out my recipe for Chinese poached chicken on page 161. It's totally O.M.G. good!

Re-program your tastebuds

I need to tell you that if you have been living off junk food or smothering your meat and vegies in oily, fatty, salty and sugary sauces and toppings, then your tastebuds are now, without a doubt, working against you.

For those of you who say, 'I don't eat junk food/fast food so I'm okay', think again. Sugar and salt is in every type of processed food, and in unbelievable quantities. What this means is that our tastebuds are overstimulated to the point of desensitisation and need more and more sweet and salty food to register 'taste'.

This unfortunately can start in childhood, when *everything* must be salted or sweetened (tomato sauce anyone?). Not only will these foods stunt the development of a child's palate, creating an addiction to salt and sugar, but also send them to the land of the overweight.

With sugar and salt, the more you get the more you want and the less you'll want to eat healthy fresh food because it doesn't seem to taste as good. But thankfully you *can* change this. I have to be honest and say that this takes time, up to four weeks or more, but you can re-program your tastebuds to appreciate the subtler flavours of wholefood. And it will be worth it. You'll not only be rescuing your tastebuds, but also reducing the size of your gut, helping your brain, boosting your energy levels, and saving money.

One way to help re-program your tastebuds is to use naturally flavoursome ingredients rather than sugar and salt. I always use fresh herbs in my cooking, and zingy vegies like onion, garlic, chilli and ginger feature in most of my recipes. I buy one or two different fresh herbs each week and keep them in the fridge in an airtight container lined with a piece of paper towel so they last the distance. For leafy herbs like coriander and parsley, I stand them in a tall glass with an inch of water in the bottom, and store them in the fridge.

Better still, start your own herb garden, with each person in your family having their own herb to care for. This is yet another way to have children become interested in food and to learn to take responsibility for what they eat. The rewards will far outweigh the effort.

As for using sauces and condiments, *read the label*. Ingredients are always listed in order of quantity from greatest to least, so if sugar or salt comes up in the first five, put the bottle back on the shelf and look for an alternative. Soy sauce is naturally salty, so go for the salt-reduced version. Most stocks and condiments come in salt-reduced versions, too, but you really must be careful with your measurements.

Hoisin can be salty and sugary. Pick one that has around 200 mg of salt (sodium) in a 20 ml tablespoon and is around 1 calorie per ml. Be vigilant with the calorie, sugar and salt content of oyster sauce and fish sauce, too, and be prepared to decrease the portion size if there are no other alternatives.

Salad dressings can turn an otherwise healthy meal into a calorie-fest. I get nervous when I see my contestants using the 'diet' dressings. Even if the dressing is low in fat, sugar, salt and calories, the old 'heavy hand' usually comes into play and they can no longer simply have a salad without it. I prefer to use the occasional splash of red wine vinegar or a little balsamic, but will often have a salad with just cracked pepper and lemon juice. Yum!

If they can do it . . .

It took a lot of patience to re-program the taste buds of the contestants on *The Biggest Loser*. They were essentially detoxing (see pages 40–2), so they got headaches and mood swings. Some were consistently at me to allow certain products back into the house. Interestingly, I found it to be the younger ones, the ones who'd had junk food from a very early age, to be the most stubborn.

With every season though, once we got through the first month, attitudes changed for the better, concentration, focus and clarity kicked in as did better sleeping patterns. There were a number of reasons for this (weight loss and fitness), but it was the clean diet that started it all.

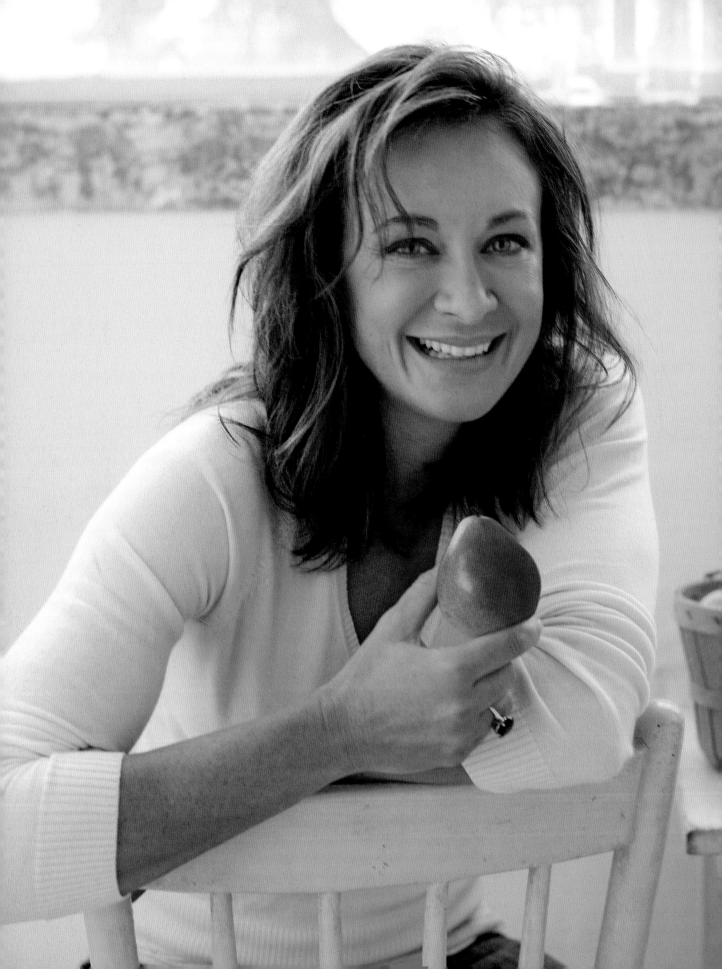

Part 2

The 12-week menu plan

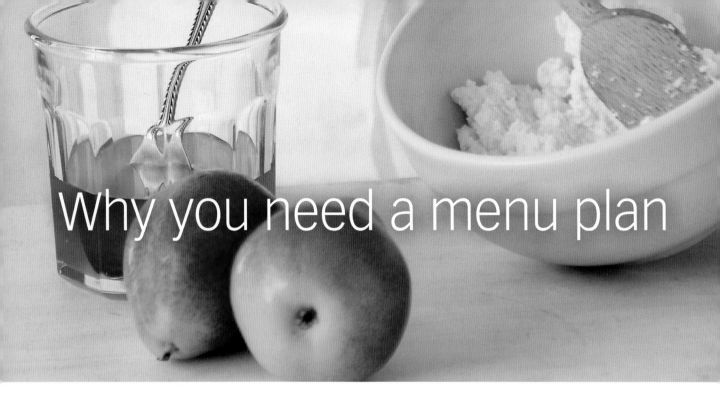

Why you need a menu plan

I always create a menu plan for my clients – it's what they expect. But first I get them to keep a seven-day food diary. This is because the first step to controlling food choices is to identify them, and my clients need to know exactly what foods (and how much of them) have led to their weight and health issues.

Even if you're fairly happy with your weight, I'd recommend that you complete a food diary – you may get a few surprises. The golden rule is: *do not diet*. It must be a full and honest account of everything you've eaten and drunk every day for a week, plus the calories. I make it very clear to my clients that if they are overweight and they come to me with a food diary that reads like Mother Teresa's I will beat them over the head with it and tell them to stop wasting everyone's time! It's of no value if it doesn't acknowledge the truth.

Once my clients have completed an honest seven-day food diary, and can *see* from their calorie counts just why they are overweight, I give them a new menu plan which gives them a set calorie quota for each day – and *they stick to it*! I usually set my girls on 1200–1350 calories per day and my guys on 1300–1600 calories per day. The range allows for differences in age, weight, height, and activity levels. It also allows for minor variations in meals and snacks during the day. Most people don't need any more than this unless they are particularly active, in which case they probably won't be overweight anyway. Trust me, there's a good reason why you don't see too many obese manual labourers!

For clients who really need help to shift their weight, I don't include a weekly 'treat' meal (where they eat a favourite meal with dessert and alcohol). If you fall into this category, don't have treat meals. You'll not only lose weight faster, but will also benefit from disciplining yourself to say 'no'. It's time to let go of sugary, fatty foods for a while. Not forever, just for a while. It's this discipline which gives you back control. Many of my clients actually tell me that they don't even want a treat meal. They already know that this type of food is the reason they are in trouble.

Your calorie quotas

If you only want to lose a couple of kilos, or want to maintain your weight, your quotas can be slightly higher than the ones I use with my clients: 1200–1500 calories for girls (three meals each at around 300–350 calories plus one or two snacks at around 100–150), and 1300–1800 calories for guys (three meals each at around 400–450 calories plus one or two snacks at around 200 calories).

As you can see, there's not a lot of difference between the quota for weight loss and the quota for weight management – only 150–200 calories. That's because once you've reached your goal weight, you can never go back to your old eating habits. You're an average-sized person now, and this is how normal people eat.

But how do you stick to the calorie quotas? This is where the menu plan comes in. I have mixed and matched my delicious recipes from Part 3, which are *all* low in calories and high in nutrition. Each breakfast, lunch and dinner recipe is designed to be less than 350 calories per

Remember – the calorie count is the key to weight control.

serve, so by adding in a snack or two from the snack section (less than 150 calories each) your daily quota will be around 1200–1350. Guys will need to bump up their calories by adding a serve of rice, pasta, or a slice of wholegrain bread.

If you have got some weight to shift, my menu plan will see you losing 1–3 per cent of your body weight per week, depending on your exercise routine and your incidental activity. This is because the plan will put you in calorie deficit, instead of the calorie surplus that you're in now.

How to use the plan

The most important thing to remember is that this menu plan isn't gospel. There will be some recipes you love, and some recipes that, well, just won't appeal to you. For example, you may be allergic to fish, or not a big fan of lentils. If so, simply swap meals – there are plenty of recipes to choose from. You might also prefer to have the same breakfast every morning for a week, and then splash out with a cooked breakfast over the weekend. The great thing is that you will always know how many calories you are taking on board, as I have calculated these for every meal. Remember – the calorie count is the key to weight control.

You'll also notice that there are never more than three red-meat dishes per week. I love red meat, but I'm careful with how much I eat and you should be too. Diets high in red meat have been linked with intestinal cancers such as bowel and colon, as they are not only high in saturated fat but frequently low in fibre. Kangaroo, however, is on a par with white fish when it comes to fat, cholesterol and calories. It really is a super food, so I often use it instead of beef in my recipes.

There are lots of vegetarian meals in the plan. In fact, there's at least one every day. You'll be amazed by how many vegetables you can eat for just a handful of calories, so I don't want to hear 'It's not enough, I'm going to be hungry!' You won't.

By the end of the twelve weeks you'll know exactly which dishes you love, and you'll not only be good at cooking them, but also be confident that they are always healthy and calorie controlled.

As you know, I'm a big fan of 'efficient' cooking – making extra to be re-used later – and I've included those kinds of meals on the weekend for the first couple of weeks until you get used to cooking up a storm. I've also left the meals that take longer to cook for the weekends or Friday nights, particularly in the first few weeks. The leftovers from these meals will be used for lunches. When cooking spag bol, for example, I get you to cook up extra portions to freeze. These can be warmed up on toast for a winter's lunch, served on some steamed bok choy for a light meal, or used as a base for a quick chilli con carne (just add beans). Now we're talking!

Bigger lunches, smaller dinners

You'll notice that a lot of the lunches are leftovers because this cookbook is not only about helping you lose weight, but also about saving you time and money. Being creatures of habit, many of us prefer to have the same thing for lunch every day, which is fine, provided we know the calorie count. But if you buy a daily sambo, do the sums: an average $8.50 sandwich five days a week will cost you over $2000 a year! My sandwiches and wraps (pages 76–83) are a tastier and cheaper option.

As for the dinners, these will probably be less than you're used to eating in the evening. This is intentional! High-calorie meals at night sluiced down with a couple of glasses of wine will fast track you to a big butt! Also, you don't want to go to bed feeling full – you're not going to be burning any of those extra calories while you're sleeping. If anything, you need to slip yourself between the sheets looking forward to a hearty breakfast. Remember – take on the energy when you're going to need it.

Catering for a family

I often hear people, particularly mums, say they are overweight because the rest of the

Tips for recipe variations

Once you've mastered a particular recipe, you might want to experiment – substituting different vegetables or different meats. For example, you might want to try kangaroo instead of beef for the Thai beef salad (page 104) which would bring the calorie count down on this recipe. Or you might want to have the lentil and cumin mash (page 185) with the mustard steak (page 173) instead of the kangaroo. Just make sure that when you vary your ingredients, you are not exceeding your daily calorie limits.

In our house we have around five breakfast and seven evening meals that we use a lot. But we don't always cook them with the same ingredients: it depends on what's in season. The best example of this would have to be stir-fries. My husband Billy is a stir-fry master and the vegies are always served up crisp and delicious. But sometimes we might be out of green beans, so we'll use asparagus or broccolini instead. Or we may be all out of coriander but we've got some lemongrass in the fridge.

When you're learning to mix and match, use the following as a guide:

- **Asian-style:** coriander, basil, lemongrass, chilli, garlic, ginger, mint, oyster mushrooms, shiitake mushrooms, baby corn, bean shoots, choy sum, bok choy, snake beans, shallots, capsicum, onion
- **Italian-style:** basil, oregano, thyme, mixed dried herbs, Italian (flat-leaf) parsley, pepper, tabasco, lemon zest, garlic, tomato, eggplant, capsicum, mushrooms, capers, olives, parmesan cheese, ricotta cheese
- **Traditional soups and casseroles:** bay leaves, rosemary, thyme, sage, Worcestershire sauce, garlic, onion, shallots, leeks, celery

family like to eat the kind of food that they should be avoiding. Well hear this: *all* of my recipes are 'family proof'! For example, spaghetti bolognese is a favourite that regularly turns up on Australian tables. To keep the calories down, simply serve the sauce on a plate of steamed greens and let the rest of the family tuck into the pasta version. For stir-fries, stick to the portions in the recipe to keep *your* weight in check, but for your growing children and teenagers, or to bump up the calorie quota for any manual workers in the house, cook some rice – half a cup of cooked long-grain white or brown rice adds about 110 calories.

Don't forget your snacks

My menu plan doesn't tell you which snacks to eat on which days for several reasons. Firstly, you may decide you don't want snacks at all. This is fine, especially if you have some weight to shift. Just be careful, though, that you don't get so hungry that you make poor food choices. Secondly, snack choices are very individual – some people are happy with an apple at 3 p.m. each afternoon, while others like to have something different every day. I give you lots of yummy snack ideas on pages 198–205. Just make sure you include them in your daily calorie counts. Girls don't want their daily quotas to go above 1500 calories and boys should stick to less than 1800.

Week 1

When you see a ♨ symbol it means you'll be preparing extra for another meal. A ✓ symbol means you'll be using leftovers. I've tried to organise leftovers to be re-used in 1–3 days, but in a couple of instances you will need to freeze them.

Tip – Don't forget to add in one or two snacks per day if you need them (pages 198-205) and include them in your totals.

	Breakfast	Lunch	Dinner	Total cals
Monday	Oat porridge with berries, p. 51 268 cal	Salad sandwich, p. 82 310 cal	♨ Minestrone, p. 70 294 cal	872
Tuesday	Fruit and muesli, p. 52 359 cal	✓ Minestrone, p. 70 294 cal	Kangaroo with watercress, chickpea, tomato and basil salad, p. 109 341 cal	994
Wednesday	Cottage cheese toast with tomato and rocket, p. 54 283 cal	Smoked salmon and avocado wrap with watercress, p. 82 318 cal	♨ Ratatouille, p. 116 247 cal	848
Thursday	Bran and mixed berries with banana, p. 52 340 cal	✓ Ratatouille, p. 116 247 cal	Chicken with fennel, cabbage, radish and cranberry coleslaw, p. 94 290 cal	877
Friday	Spiced pear and ricotta toast, p. 57 353 cal	Chilli beef stir-fry, p. 178 323 cal	Zesty tofu and shiitake mushroom stir-fry, p. 118 295 cal	971
Saturday	Poached eggs on garlic toast with wilted spinach, p. 67 290 cal	Wholemeal penne with zucchini, lemon zest and parsley, p. 128 356 cal	Lamb and sweet potato tagine, p. 163 296 cal + Ginger and lime fruit salad, p. 193 110 cal	1052
Sunday	Beans on toast with fried egg, p. 62 360 cal	Chicken salad with baby spinach, blackberries, apple, feta and walnut, p. 98 348 cal	♨ Lentil, leek and mushroom loaf, p. 129 261 cal	969

Weekly total **6583**

Plus snacks _____

Week 2

The breakfast options are just suggestions. If you're like me, you'll probably have the same breakfast on weekdays (I have porridge or muesli) and save the cooked brekkies for the weekends.

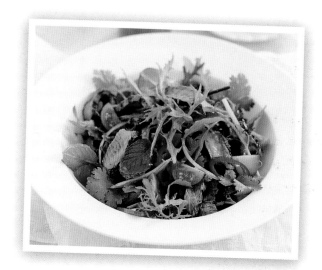

	Breakfast	Lunch	Dinner	Total cals
Monday	Fruit and muesli, p. 52 359 cal	Mediterranean sandwich with olive and basil tapenade, p. 79 176 cal	🍲 Thai beef salad, p. 104 225 cal	760
Tuesday	Cottage cheese toast with tomato and rocket, p. 54 283 cal	✓ Roast beef sandwich, p. 81 317 cal	Grilled capsicum and zucchini pizza with feta, p. 127 314 cal	914
Wednesday	Beans on toast with fried egg, p. 62 360 cal	✓ Lentil, leek and mushroom loaf, p. 129 261 cal	Zucchini, green bean and beef stir-fry with hoisin sauce, p. 176 300 cal	886
Thursday	Spiced pear and ricotta toast, p. 57 353 cal	Salad sandwich, p. 82 310 cal	Char-grilled vegetable terrine, p. 111 221 cal	884
Friday	Bran and mixed berries with banana, p. 52 340 cal	Mixed herb, ricotta and tomato wrap, p. 81 214 cal	Chicken sang choy bow, p. 157 248 cal	802
Saturday	Oat porridge with berries, p. 51 268 cal	Spicy Cajun chicken kebabs with mixed leaf salad, p. 148 286 cal	🍲 Lentil shepherd's pie with steamed broccoli, p. 115 290 cal + Baked pears and ricotta with honey, sultanas and cinnamon, p. 197 107 cal	951
Sunday	Egg-white omelette with garlic mushrooms, p. 61 300 cal	Tom yum soup with rice crackers, p. 75 129 cal	🍲 Salmon patties with tomato salsa, p. 133 339 cal	768

Weekly total   **5965**
Plus snacks   _____

Week 3

Even if you only need to lose a few kilos, it's a good idea to see if you can go without Saturday's dessert for the first few weeks. You'll feel empowered, and find it much easier to make healthy food choices.

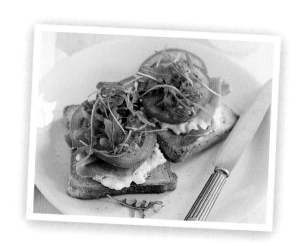

	Breakfast	Lunch	Dinner	Total cals
Monday	Cottage cheese toast with tomato and rocket, p. 54 283 cal	Niçoise salad, p. 92 265 cal	Chicken rice paper rolls, p. 159 333 cal	881
Tuesday	Bran and mixed berries with banana, p. 52 340 cal	✔ Lentil shepherd's pie with steamed broccoli, p. 115 290 cal	Char-grilled chicken with tomato salsa, p. 154 321 cal	951
Wednesday	Spiced pear and ricotta toast, p. 57 353 cal	Salad sandwich, p. 82 310 cal	Cauliflower, spinach and ricotta bake, p. 124 244 cal	907
Thursday	Fruit and muesli, p. 52 359 cal	✔ Salmon patties with tomato salsa, p. 133 339 cal	Roast kangaroo with lentil and cumin mash, p. 185 317 cal	1015
Friday	Oat porridge with berries, p. 51 268 cal	🥣 Pumpkin soup, p. 69 227 cal	Thai green chicken curry, p. 150 368 cal	863
Saturday	Beans on toast with fried egg, p. 62 360 cal	Cumin-crusted lamb cutlets with lemony broccoli and broad beans, p. 167 321 cal	Stir-fried snapper with shallots, broccolini and shiitake mushrooms, p. 140 335 cal + Poached rhubarb with yoghurt and basil, p. 188 103 cal	1119
Sunday	Whole-egg omelette with corn, spinach and dill, p. 58 389 cal	Zucchini, green bean and mint risotto, p. 125 361 cal	🥣 Roast beef and vegetables, p. 181 309 cal	1059

Weekly total 6795
Plus snacks _____

Week 4

I'm a big fan of efficient cooking. This week features three recipes where you cook extra for other meals.

	Breakfast	Lunch	Dinner	Total cals
Monday	Bran and mixed berries with banana, p. 52 340 cal	✓ Roast beef sandwich, p. 81 317 cal	🥢 Chinese poached chicken, p. 161 268 cal	925
Tuesday	Beans on toast with fried egg, p. 62 325 cal	✓ Pumpkin soup, p. 69 227 cal	Vegetable stacks with tofu, p. 117 341 cal	893
Wednesday	Fruit and muesli, p. 52 359 cal	Mediterranean sandwich with olive and basil tapenade, p. 79 176 cal	Salmon with tartare sauce and rocket salad, p. 89 288 cal	823
Thursday	Oat porridge with berries, p. 51 310 cal	✓ Chicken, eggplant and hummus sandwich, p. 78 276 cal	Mixed vegetable stir-fry with oyster sauce, p. 120 239 cal	825
Friday	Cottage cheese toast with tomato and rocket, p. 54 283 cal	Rocket, grape, walnut and parmesan salad, p. 87 258 cal	Tomato, anchovy and basil pizza, p. 136 307 cal	848
Saturday	Scrambled eggs with grilled asparagus and tomatoes, p. 64 335 cal	Salmon with char-grilled asparagus and tomato salad, p. 90 269 cal	🥢 Zucchini, eggplant and mushroom lasagne, p. 122 229 cal + Strawberry and passionfruit yoghurt semifreddo, p. 190 103 cal	936
Sunday	Spiced pear and ricotta toast, p. 57 353 cal	Beef and ramen noodle soup, p. 72 351 cal	🥢 Roast lemon and oregano chicken with mixed vegetables, p. 145 339 cal	1043

Weekly total   **6293**

Plus snacks   _____

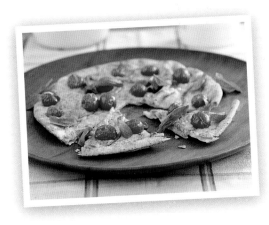

Week 5

This weekend you aren't making anything for leftovers, but feel free to make more of the risoni or chicken parcels on Saturday so that you will have something ready for lunch next week.

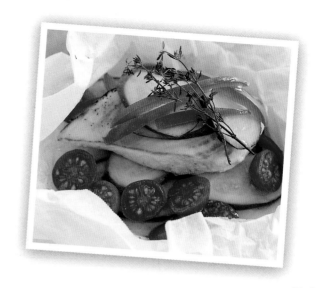

	Breakfast	Lunch	Dinner	Total cals
Monday	Fruit and muesli, p. 52 359 cal	✔ Chicken and avocado sandwich, p. 76 300 cal	Zesty tofu and shiitake mushroom stir-fry, p. 118 295 cal	954
Tuesday	Bran and mixed berries with banana, p. 52 340 cal	Tabbouleh, p. 86 227 cal	Kangaroo and mint salad with char-grilled zucchini and capsicum, p. 106 276 cal	843
Wednesday	Cottage cheese toast with tomato and rocket, p. 54 283 cal	✔ Zucchini, eggplant and mushroom lasagne, p. 122 229 cal	Grilled capsicum and zucchini pizza with feta, p. 127 314 cal	826
Thursday	Oat porridge with berries, p. 51 268 cal	Salad sandwich, p. 82 310 cal	Barbecued ginger and lemon prawns, p. 142 195 cal	773
Friday	Egg-white omelette with garlic mushrooms, p. 61 300 cal	Open beef burgers, p. 168 256 cal	Baby beet, chickpea, basil and feta salad, p. 85 327 cal	883
Saturday	Beans on toast with fried egg, p. 62 360 cal	Risoni, tuna, baby spinach and snowpea salad with lemon and dill, p. 93 304 cal	Mediterranean chicken parcels, p. 158 316 cal + Berry jelly, p. 194 99 cal	1079
Sunday	Poached eggs on garlic toast with wilted spinach, p. 67 290 cal	Tom yum soup with rice crackers, p. 75 129 cal	Baked fish and chips, p. 131 362 cal	781

Weekly total   **6139**

Plus snacks   _____

Week 6

This week features heaps of efficient cooking! Cook extra of the leek and asparagus soup on Monday to use for a weekday lunch.

Tip – Freeze leftovers of the lentil, leek and mushroom loaf and the spicy beef and vegetable meatloaf.

	Breakfast	Lunch	Dinner	Total cals
Monday	Bran and mixed berries with banana, p. 52 340 cal	Smoked salmon and avocado wrap with watercress, p. 82 318 cal	☕ Leek and asparagus soup, p. 71 166 cal	824
Tuesday	Whole-egg omelette with corn, spinach and dill, p. 58 389 cal	Salad sandwich, p. 82 310 cal	Tuna kebabs, p. 142 319 cal	1018
Wednesday	Cottage cheese toast with tomato and rocket, p. 54 283 cal	Mediterranean sandwich with olive and basil tapenade, p. 79 176 cal	☕ Lentil, leek and mushroom loaf, p. 129 261 cal	720
Thursday	Oat porridge with berries, p. 51 268 cal	✓ Leek and asparagus soup, p. 71 166 cal	Lamb and sweet potato tagine, p. 163 296 cal	730
Friday	Fruit and muesli, p. 52 359 cal	Seafood linguini, p. 135 377 cal	☕ Spicy beef and vegetable meatloaf, p. 174 265 cal	1001
Saturday	Scrambled eggs with grilled asparagus and tomatoes, p. 64 335 cal	Rocket, grape, walnut and parmesan salad, p. 87 258 cal	☕ Chicken and vegetable soup with silverbeet, p. 74 317 cal + Lemon mousse, p. 187 102 cal	1012
Sunday	Spiced pear and ricotta toast, p. 57 353 cal	Chicken pad thai, p. 153 344 cal	☕ Tuna mornay, p. 139 317 cal	1014

Weekly total 6319

Plus snacks _____

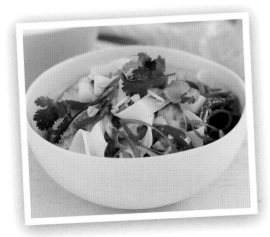

Week 7

Beans are a super food – packed with protein, low-GI carbs and vitamins. Use the extra beans from Sunday's brekkie to make beans on toast for Monday's lunch.

> Tip – Freeze enough spag bol sauce leftovers for two more lunches.

	Breakfast	Lunch	Dinner	Total cals
Monday	Cottage cheese toast with tomato and rocket, p. 54 283 cal	✔ Lentil, leek and mushroom loaf, p. 129 261 cal	Mixed vegetable stir-fry with oyster sauce, p. 120 239 cal	783
Tuesday	Bran and mixed berries with banana, p. 52 340 cal	✔ Tuna mornay, p. 139 317 cal	Kangaroo with watercress, chickpea, tomato and basil salad, p. 109 341 cal	998
Wednesday	Spiced pear and ricotta toast, p. 57 353 cal	Smoked salmon and avocado wrap with watercress, p. 82 318 cal	Mixed vegetable and tofu stir-fry, p. 119 291 cal	962
Thursday	Fruit and muesli, p. 52 359 cal	✔ Chicken and vegetable soup with silverbeet, p. 74 317 cal	Roasted vegetables and tofu with rosemary, p. 112 343 cal	1019
Friday	Oat porridge with berries, p. 51 268 cal	Salad sandwich, p. 82 310 cal	⬮ Spaghetti bolognese, p. 170 422 cal	1000
Saturday	Whole-egg omelette with corn, spinach and dill, p. 58 389 cal	Cauliflower, spinach and ricotta bake, p. 124 244 cal	Lamb shanks with green beans and mushrooms, p. 164 329 cal + Baked pears and ricotta with honey, sultanas and cinnamon, p. 197 107 cal	1069
Sunday	⬮ Beans on toast with fried egg, p. 62 360 cal	Spicy stir-fried prawns with snowpeas, asparagus and wombok, p. 143 291 cal	⬮ Ratatouille, p. 116 247 cal	898

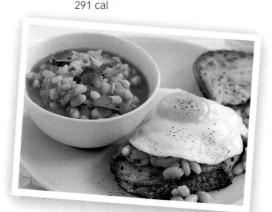

Weekly total 6729
Plus snacks ____

Week 8

By now you'll be feeling so much more confident in the kitchen! I'm hoping you'll even be experimenting. Go for it!

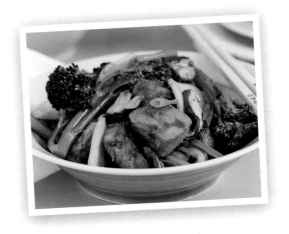

	Breakfast	Lunch	Dinner	Total cals
Monday	Oat porridge with berries, p. 51 268 cal	✔ Beans on toast, p. 62 265 cal	☲ Minestrone, p. 70 294 cal	827
Tuesday	Fruit and muesli, p. 52 359 cal	✔ Ratatouille, p. 116 247 cal	Kanga Bangas with sweet potato mash, p. 183 347 cal	953
Wednesday	Cottage cheese toast with tomato and rocket, p. 54 283 cal	Smoked salmon and avocado wrap with watercress, p. 82 318 cal	Grilled capsicum and zucchini pizza with feta, p. 127 314 cal	915
Thursday	Bran and mixed berries with banana, p. 52 340 cal	✔ Minestrone, p. 70 294 cal	Chicken with fennel, cabbage, radish and cranberry coleslaw, p. 94 290 cal	924
Friday	Spiced pear and ricotta toast, p. 57 353 cal	✔ Spaghetti bolognese, p. 170 422 cal	Zesty tofu and shiitake mushroom stir-fry, p. 118 295 cal	1070
Saturday	Poached eggs on garlic toast with wilted spinach, p. 67 290 cal	Wholemeal penne with zucchini, lemon zest and parsley, p. 128 356 cal	Mustard steak with steamed vegies, p. 173 313 cal + Strawberry and passionfruit yoghurt semifreddo, p. 190 103 cal	1062
Sunday	Beans on toast with fried egg, p. 62 360 cal	Chicken salad with baby spinach, blackberries, apple, feta and walnut, p. 98 348 cal	Chinese steamed trevalla with baby bok choy, p. 138 233 cal	941

Weekly total 6692

Plus snacks _____

Week 9

Prepare a little extra beef for Monday's Thai beef salad, and use the lovely thin slices for a tasty beef sandwich on Tuesday.

> Tip – Don't forget to add in any snacks to each day's calorie totals.

	Breakfast	Lunch	Dinner	Total cals
Monday	Fruit and muesli, p. 52 359 cal	Mediterranean sandwich with olive and basil tapenade, p. 79 176 cal	🥢 Thai beef salad, p. 104 225 cal	760
Tuesday	Cottage cheese toast with tomato and rocket, p. 54 283 cal	✔ Roast beef sandwich, p. 81 317 cal	Grilled capsicum and zucchini pizza with feta, p. 127 314 cal	914
Wednesday	Beans on toast with fried egg, p. 62 360 cal	Mixed herb, ricotta and tomato wrap, p. 81 214 cal	Chicken sang choy bow, p. 157 248 cal	822
Thursday	Spiced pear and ricotta toast, p. 57 353 cal	Salad sandwich, p. 82 310 cal	Stir-fried snapper with shallots, broccolini and shiitake mushrooms, p. 140 335 cal	998
Friday	Bran and mixed berries with banana, p. 52 340 cal	Rocket, grape, walnut and parmesan salad, p. 87 258 cal	Roasted vegetables and tofu with rosemary, p. 112 343 cal	941
Saturday	Oat porridge with berries, p. 51 268 cal	Spicy Cajun chicken kebabs with mixed leaf salad, p. 148 286 cal	Char-grilled vegetable terrine, p. 111 221 cal + Lemon mousse, p. 187 102 cal	877
Sunday	Egg-white omelette with garlic mushrooms, p. 61 300 cal	Lamb, cannellini bean and rocket salad, p. 103 312 cal	Thai chicken stir-fry, p. 147 315 cal	927

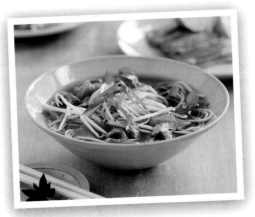

Weekly total 6239
Plus snacks _____

Week 10

For even more efficient cooking, double the portions in Tuesday's chicken with tomato salsa. This leaves you with enough for two more lunches, or three if you serve each portion wrapped in a slice of wholemeal mountain bread.

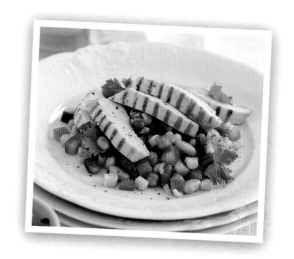

	Breakfast	Lunch	Dinner	Total cals
Monday	Cottage cheese toast with tomato and rocket, p. 54 283 cal	Mixed herb, ricotta and tomato wrap, p. 81 214 cal	⬆ Chicken and vegetable soup with silverbeet, p. 74 317 cal	814
Tuesday	Bran and mixed berries with banana, p. 52 340 cal	✓ Chicken and vegetable soup with silverbeet, p. 74 317 cal	⬆ Char-grilled chicken with tomato salsa, p. 154 321 cal	978
Wednesday	Spiced pear and ricotta toast, p. 57 353 cal	✓ Char-grilled chicken with tomato salsa, p. 154 321 cal	Cauliflower, spinach and ricotta bake, p. 124 244 cal	918
Thursday	Fruit and muesli, p. 52 359 cal	Salad sandwich, p. 82 310 cal	Roast kangaroo with lentil and cumin mash, p. 185 317 cal	986
Friday	Oat porridge with berries, p. 51 268 cal	✓ Spaghetti bolognese, p. 170 422 cal	⬆ Lentil shepherd's pie with steamed broccoli, p. 115 290 cal	980
Saturday	Beans on toast with fried egg, p. 62 360 cal	Buckwheat noodle salad with sesame seeds, p. 86 353 cal	Whole baked snapper with fennel, onion and tomato, p. 132 328 cal + Poached rhubarb with yoghurt and basil, p. 188 103 cal	956
Sunday	Whole-egg omelette with corn, spinach and dill, p. 58 389 cal	✓ Lentil shepherd's pie with steamed broccoli, p. 115 290 cal	⬆ Roast beef and vegetables, p. 181 309 cal	988

Weekly total 6620
Plus snacks _____

Week 11

Use some leftovers from Monday night's poached chicken to make Tuesday's sandwich. Don't forget to add in your snacks.

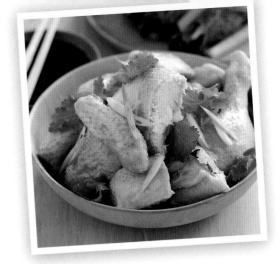

	Breakfast	Lunch	Dinner	Total cals
Monday	Bran and mixed berries with banana, p. 52 340 cal	✔ Roast beef sandwich, p. 81 317 cal	☕ Chinese poached chicken, p. 161 268 cal	925
Tuesday	Beans on toast with fried egg, p. 62 360 cal	✔ Chicken, eggplant and hummus sandwich, p. 78 275 cal	Mixed vegetable and tofu stir-fry, p. 119 291 cal	926
Wednesday	Fruit and muesli, p. 52 359 cal	Mediterranean sandwich with olive and basil tapenade, p. 79 176 cal	Salmon with tartare sauce and rocket salad, p. 89 288 cal	823
Thursday	Oat porridge with berries, p. 51 268 cal	Salad sandwich, p. 82 310 cal	Chicken with fennel, cabbage, radish and cranberry coleslaw, p. 94 290 cal	868
Friday	Cottage cheese toast with tomato and rocket, p. 57 283 cal	Beef and ramen noodle soup, p. 72 351 cal	Tomato, anchovy and basil pizza, p. 136 307 cal	941
Saturday	Spiced pear and ricotta toast, p. 57 353 cal	Salmon with char-grilled asparagus and tomato salad, p. 90 269 cal	Vegetable stacks with tofu, p. 117 341 cal + Ginger and lime fruit salad, p. 193 110 cal	1073
Sunday	Scrambled eggs with grilled asparagus and tomatoes, p. 64 335 cal	Zucchini, green bean and mint risotto, p. 125 361 cal	☕ Roast lemon and oregano chicken with mixed vegetables, p. 145 339 cal	1035

Weekly total   **6591**
Plus snacks   _____

Week 12

Congratulations! You've made it to Week 12.

You've taken control in the kitchen and are in charge of your weight, your health, and your life!

	Breakfast	Lunch	Dinner	Total cals
Monday	Fruit and muesli, p. 52 359 cal	✓ Chicken and avocado sandwich, p. 76 300 cal	≋ Zucchini, eggplant and mushroom lasagne, p. 122 229 cal	888
Tuesday	Bran and mixed berries with banana, p. 52 340 cal	Mixed herb, ricotta and tomato wrap, p. 81 214 cal	Kangaroo and mint salad with char-grilled zucchini and capsicum, p. 106 276 cal	830
Wednesday	Cottage cheese toast with tomato and rocket, p. 57 283 cal	✓ Zucchini, eggplant and mushroom lasagne, p. 122 229 cal	Risoni, tuna, baby spinach and snowpea salad with lemon and dill, p. 93 265 cal	777
Thursday	Oat porridge with berries, p. 51 268 cal	Salad sandwich, p. 82 310 cal	Barbecued ginger and lemon prawns, p. 142 195 cal	773
Friday	Egg-white omelette with garlic mushrooms, p. 61 300 cal	Open beef burgers, p. 168 256 cal	Baby beet, chickpea, basil and feta salad, p. 85 327 cal	883
Saturday	Beans on toast with fried egg, p. 62 360 cal	Grilled capsicum and zucchini pizza with feta, p. 127 314 cal	Moroccan chicken, orange and mint salad, p. 97 266 cal + Berry jelly, p. 194 99 cal	1039
Sunday	Poached eggs on garlic toast with wilted spinach, p. 67 290 cal	Salmon patties with tomato salsa, p. 133 339 cal	Baked fish and chips, p. 131 362 cal	991

Weekly total   6181
Plus snacks   _____

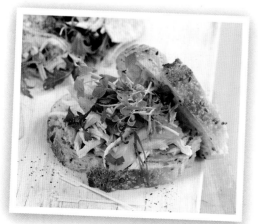

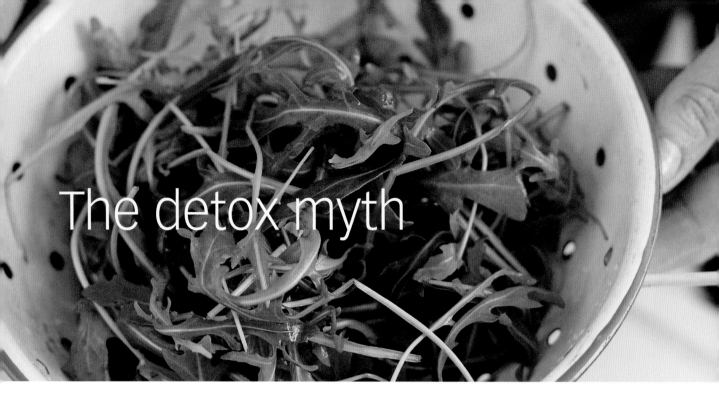

The detox myth

Despite our best efforts, human nature dictates that at times we all find ourselves gradually sliding into an unhealthy lifestyle. Whatever the reason for the lapse, we know that we are looking and feeling crap and that we need to give our bodies a break.

Now I have to admit that I don't really like the word 'detox' or even the word 'cleansing' (especially when it accompanies the word 'diet'). These are misleading and suggest that we are 'dirty' and that we have accumulated chemicals that can only be removed by expensive pills, elixirs or procedures. Thankfully we were equipped at birth with the greatest detoxifier the planet has ever known – our bodies, and all we need to do is to take some of the workload off our organs by giving them less to do.

As well as cutting out the 'baddies' and pumping up the 'goodies' (see the lists below) I

make sure I'm getting eight hours uninterrupted sleep every night. Sometimes I cut out or reduce bread, red meat, some white meat and dairy for short spells, too, as these labour my digestive system. But I still make sure I get plenty of protein in my diet through fish, tofu or lentils. I've spent too many hours in the gym to give away my hard-earned muscle, and that means getting enough protein to support it, plus sufficient high-quality carbohydrates like fruit, vegetables, lentils and brown rice to keep my energy levels up for my training.

Many so-called detox diets are nothing more than high-glucose diets, which will keep your brain functioning but at the expense of your muscle tissue. You'll lose weight because you'll lose fat, but you'll also lose muscle. As soon as the 'detox' is over, you'll go back to your old habits and lifestyle and your body will put the weight back on again. However, it will be *all fat*. That's how you can end up fatter than when you started. Once that muscle is gone, you gotta work damn hard to get it back.

If you follow my 12-Week Menu Plan (or simply mix and match the recipes but stick to the calorie quotas), you are effectively 'detoxing'. Not only will you be knocking out salty, sugary, fatty, processed foods, but you'll be bumping up fresh wholefoods, with all their protein, fibre, antioxidants and other amazing nutrients.

And if you don't drink more than two nights a week and don't smoke, you're giving your body an even better headstart to health.

Cut out the baddies

1. No tobacco

If you're a smoker, then you have a 50/50 chance of dying from lung, throat or other smoking-related cancer or, if you're lucky, lugging around an oxygen bottle with a tube up your nose for the rest of your life. Think about it – if you *and* your husband/wife/mum/dad smoke, there's an even greater chance that one of you will have to watch the other die slowly in hospital from a tobacco-related illness. Nice.

2. No alcohol

We're a nation of drinkers, and the research tells us that we're doing more of it. Yet the long-term effects can be devastating: sleep, memory and concentration difficulties; heart, brain and liver damage; and an increased risk of cancer. If you think, 'Yeah, well I don't drink excessively', take a measuring cup and measure out 150 ml of wine into a wine glass, otherwise known as one standard drink for a female. It's rather sobering. Take alcohol out of your diet altogether when you're having a clean-up – you'll instantly lose weight and feel amazing. Afterwards, aim to have four or five alcohol-free days. If you find you can't go two days in a row without alcohol, you might need to ask yourself some hard questions.

3. No caffeine

This drug is everywhere – coffee, tea, chocolate, soft drinks and energy drinks – and it's not a drug you want around when you're cleaning out the body cupboards. It reduces iron absorption when you drink it with meals and messes around with your B group vitamins.

4. No sugar

Our obsession with sugar is part of the reason Australia is the fattest nation on the planet. Fructose and sucrose is in everything, including in most of our so called 'diet' products. Your diet needs to be full of wholefoods, so refined carbohydrates like sugar are a definite no-no. Read your labels!

5. No processed food

Much of the food we see in a box, tin or packet has a long shelf life, sometimes up to three years. There's a really good reason for that – sugar, salt and chemical preservatives. As mentioned above, sugar is a big problem. Our digestive systems were never designed to cope with the vast amounts of sugar we are eating, or the added preservatives and salt. Behavioural problems, obesity, diabetes, asthma, cancer and many other illnesses have been linked to food additives. By taking some or all of these products out of your diet you will be giving your digestive system a well-earned break.

Pump up the goodies

1. More water

Water's groovy because it supports our body's natural detoxifying organs – our kidneys and our liver. So it makes sense to keep ourselves well hydrated. Work on around six to eight glasses a day. Filtered or spring water is fine as it tastes better, but don't go thirsty if there's only tap water available. Don't add to our burgeoning plastic water bottle problem, either. Get one bottle, maybe an insulated one to keep it cold, and fill up from home.

2. More vegetables and fruit

These are your detox and weight-loss secret weapons. Why? Fibre! Which is why I would chuck out the fruit juice and have an orange any day of the week! Two servings of fruit a day and five servings of vegetables are the Australian targets. Before you start quivering at the prospect, you should know that a 'serving' is only half a cup of vegies, a medium-sized piece of fruit, a cup of lettuce or a cup of wilted spinach. Remember that fruit is higher in calories than vegetables so keep an eye on your quantities.

Here are a few tips to get a few more fruit and vegies into your day:

- Always have an apple or a banana with you, or cut up an apple or pear, squeeze on some lemon juice (to prevent it browning), and put it in a zip-lock bag for easy snacking on the run.
- Chopped carrots, celery, string beans and snowpeas are fantastic for an afternoon snack. Plenty of fibre, really low in calories and I just love the crunch factor!
- When eating breakfast out, ask for some wilted spinach with your poached egg.
- When you're cooking porridge, mash a banana or grate an apple into the mixture, or top your breakfast cereal or yoghurt snack with half a cup of berries.
- Flip your usual fruit and cereal ratios at breakfast. Instead of a couple of token chopped strawberries or banana on top of your cereal, sprinkle a little cereal on top of a bowl of chopped fruit. This makes the meal more fruit-based.
- If you're making sauces or marinades, add a grated zucchini.
- When you're eating out, always ask for a side order of steamed vegetables or a salad (with no dressing or with the dressing on the side) rather than bread or chips.

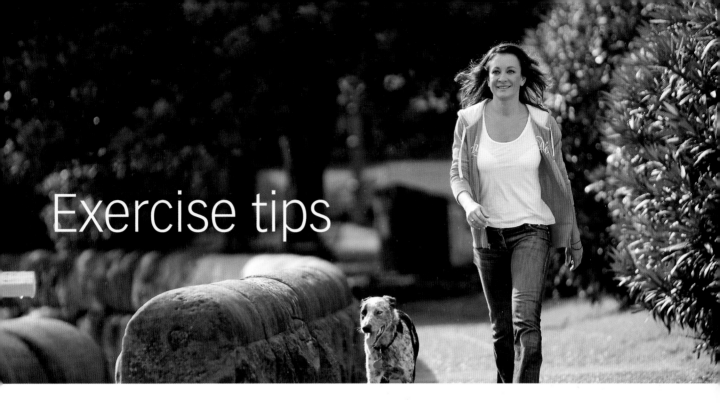

Exercise tips

In the previous chapters I explained that the key to weight management is taking control of the food you eat – preparing wholefood meals that are low in calories and high in nutrition. Now I'm here to tell you that the key to *accelerating* weight loss is exercise – put simply, the harder your heart is pumping, the more calories you're burning.

If I did no exercise at all I would burn approximately 1400 calories in 24 hours – this is my basal metabolic rate (BMR). To work out your BMR involves a fairly complicated equation with your age, weight and height, but if you log on to my website (michellebridges. com.au) the calculation will be done for you. Simply enter your details and presto!

Without exercise, I'd burn about 60 calories an hour – not much – which is why I'd still need to exercise to maintain my current weight.

There's also another reason why exercise is so great for weight loss. Exercise makes your muscles more insulin sensitive, which means your pancreas doesn't need to make as much insulin and your insulin levels drop. When there's *less* insulin in your blood to convert sugar to fat you are *less* likely to put on weight and *more* likely to lose weight if you need to.

Also, exercise decreases cortisol (a stress hormone). Cortisol can cause visceral fat deposits (fat around internal organs and tissues – think the 'beer gut' look) which are not only dangerous for your health, but are extremely hard to remove.

For these and many more reasons I encourage *all* my clients, whether they are weight-loss candidates or not, to exercise for 45–60 minutes six days a week, with three out of the six days being intense sessions, two being moderate and one being passive. It's not a perfect world and it may not always work out like that. You might have to split up a session – 20 minutes in the morning and 25 minutes in the evening, but whatever! Just get it done! See my book *Crunch Time* for a killer workout program, plus detailed descriptions of all the exercises.

My clients wear a heart-rate monitor so they can see how many calories they are burning in a session. I aim to have them blowing off at least

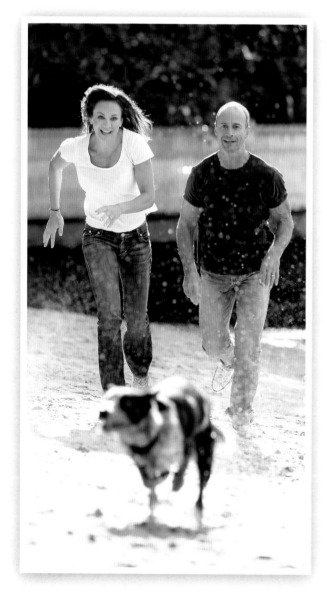

500 calories in the intense workout sessions (three per week) and to try to come close to that in the other moderate sessions.

Believe it or not, if you are looking to shed lots of weight, you need not train any harder or longer than those who are trying to maintain their weight! Why? Because the bigger you are the more calories you will expend. Some of my *Biggest Loser* contestants would burn up in 50 minutes what an average adult would burn up in three hours! However, as they got smaller and fitter it got harder to hit those big numbers, so for them 500 per session was my cut-off point.

For those of you who don't have a heart-rate monitor, the table below gives you a very rough idea of the kind of workouts that burn off around 500 calories. But I have to warn you that there is a tremendous variability in our calorie-burning abilities. Our age, gender, height, weight, muscle mass, and the type and intensity of the exercise all influence our calorie expenditure, so it's tricky to put together examples that suit everyone.

Exercise needed to burn 500 calories

	Your weight		
	70 kg	**100 kg**	**120 kg**
Brisk walk	80 min	50 min	40 min
Jog	45 min	30 min	20 min
Weights	90 min	75 min	60 min
Swim laps	50 min	40 min	30 min
Cross trainer	50 min	40 min	30 min
Boxing (hard)	40 min	25 min	20 min
Tennis	60 min	45 min	30 min

Consistency

The single most important feature of any kind of training is *consistency*. It's totally natural to feel differently about things from day to day, but you cannot use those feelings to talk yourself out of training. Don't manufacture reasons why you shouldn't exercise. Just get on with it. It's what I call 'robot mode'. Get out of bed, put on your training gear, and start your run or go to the gym *without thinking* about what you're doing.

Why? Because as soon as you blow off one training session, it's really easy to blow off the next one and then the next one until the thought of a workout churns your stomach. Before you know it, three months have passed and you've done nothing. You feel like a slug and you've put on 5 kilograms. I know because I've been there.

Exercise needs to become something you just *do* – part of everyday life. Just like you do the dishes, take out the garbage, make your bed – you exercise. It's no big deal, but the rewards are far greater than doing the dishes will ever be!

As you can see, running and other types of cardiovascular training are time-efficient, but it's important not to fall into the trap of seeing cardio training as the only way to burn calories. When using your heart-rate monitor, you'll notice that cardio training burns calories quicker than weight training, but weight training has a longer 'after-burn' effect, keeping your metabolism elevated so that you are still burning calories long after the session is over. Weight training also improves muscle insulin sensitivity, helping to keep your insulin levels down, and it tones and tightens way more than any cardio session will.

So, if you are out to burn stacks of calories in one hit, and pack on some lean muscle and get fitter, then you are better off super setting (see below under 'weights') and incorporating some basic fitness drills like jogging and boxing.

Incidental exercise plays a bigger part in all of this than you may realise, too. You've just got to keep moving. Taking the stairs, walking to work, walking home with a load of groceries, doing the house work, walking back and forth to the photocopier – it all adds up. You will get fast results when you add formal training and incidental exercise together.

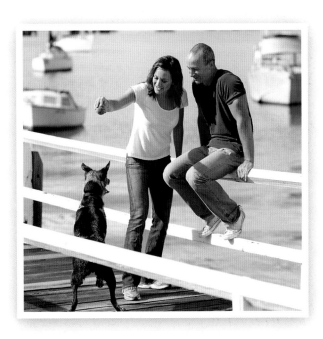

My favourite training

I'll have a go at anything, but there are a few things that I really love to do.

Group fitness classes

I am a group fitness junkie from way back, back to the days of g-string leotards and leg warmers! Classes are great and I love the fact that I get the job done in 55 minutes with fantastic music and in a group environment which has lots of energy. I love BodyPump, BodyAttack, Basic Training, Boxing, RPM and Spin. But there are plenty more to choose from. I will usually try to get there early and jump on the treadmill or cross trainer for about 15 minutes before class as a warm-up. (You can do this too if you are in the market to move some big kilos.) I have taught classes since I was fourteen, and they *rock*!

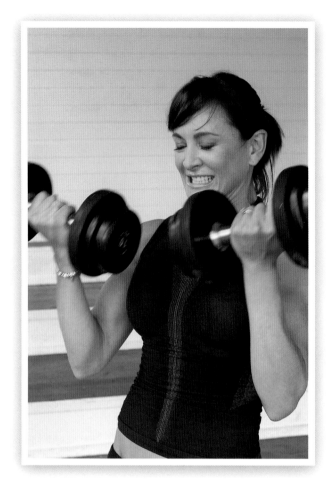

Running

Running will strip the kilos off you and improve your fitness like nothing else. I try to run at least two or three times a week, and squeeze in more if I can. It took me a few years to build up to it, but these days I make sure I grind out at least 10 kilometres each session.

If you're not a runner, start by walking at a brisk pace, with occasional periods of jogging, then gradually up the jogging periods until you are running more than you are walking. Or start with a 20-minute run – 10 minutes to a certain destination, then 10 minutes back. You'll be surprised at how quickly the gains come and your fitness improves.

Weights

You just have to push and pull things if you want to get shaped, toned and tight. Weight training is a life insurance policy. It will keep your bones strong, maintain your posture, keep your metabolism firing and allow you to continue an active life well into old age.

I do a mix of weight training workouts, BodyPump in the group fitness studio and weights in the gym. In the gym I always do super sets. These are two different exercises performed one after the other without a break, literally running from one piece of equipment to the other. When the first exercise is upper body and the second is lower body, my heart rate is slamming! There's no time for yakking in the weights room when I'm in there! Super sets are brilliant for strength, fitness and calorie expenditure. (See my book *Crunch Time* for some great weight-training exercises.) My mum started training with weights at fifty-six years of age and she's never looked back.

Boxing

After a hard day on set with my contestants there's nothing better than punching a bag till I'm dog-tired. It's liberating and releases stress like you can't imagine! And jeepers, does it burn up the calories. Try a boxing class or get a boxing coach.

Basic training circuits

These are my speciality. I put together six to eight individual exercises and I make myself do twenty repetitions of each one without stopping. I get one-minute's rest and then I repeat all of them again.

I choose a mix of upper and lower body toning exercises as well as cardiovascular exercises that really get my heart-rate up. Here's one circuit I do:

1. Basketball jumps
2. Push-ups on toes
3. Five-step sideways runs
4. Standing shoulder press with a medium barbell
5. Frog jumps holding a medicine ball
6. Over-the-fence jumps on a high bench.

The possibilities are endless. Sometimes when I'm in a really foul mood I will time myself and then on the second round I have to beat my time. I will do five or six rounds and it *smashes* the calories!

You'll find lots and lots of these circuits in my first book, *Crunch Time*. Check them out, and good luck!

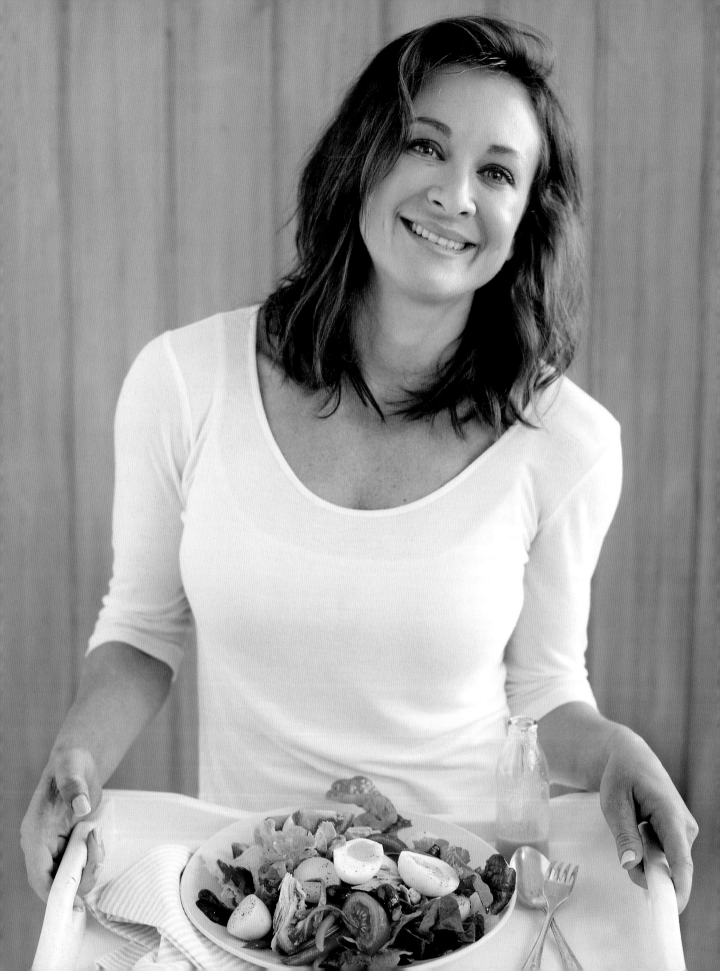

Part 3

My recipes

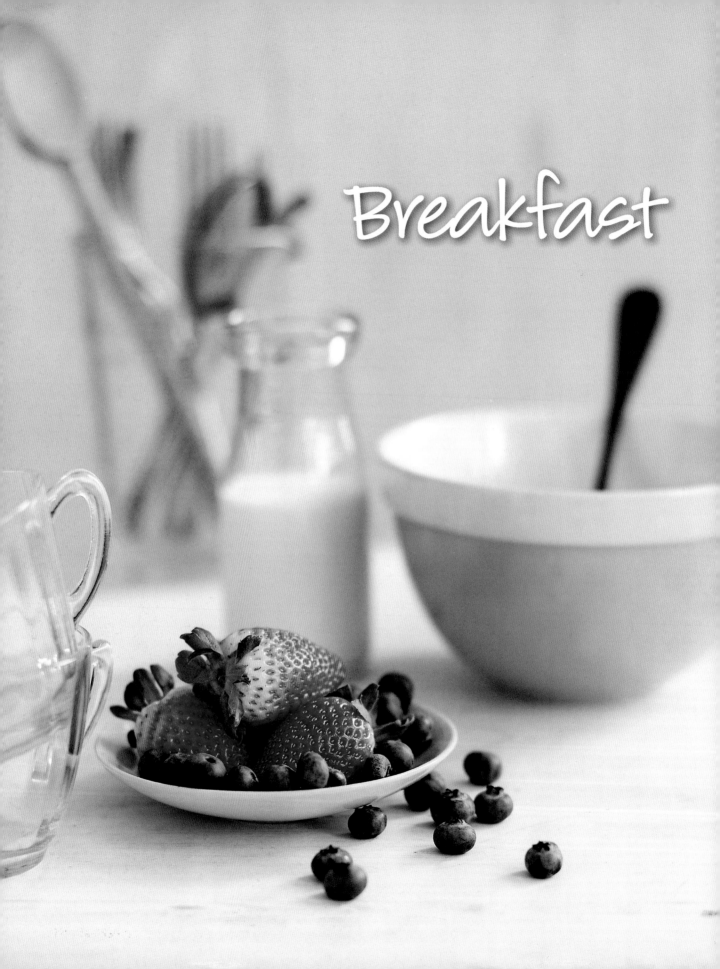

Breakfast

Oat porridge with berries

Porridge is an excellent source of low-GI carbohydrates, which give me great energy and keep me feeling fuller for longer. I love a bowl of steaming porridge on a cold morning, and with a sprinkling of berries I'm adding antioxidants *and* sweetness, with a minimum of extra calories.

Serves 2
Prep 5 minutes
Cook 15 minutes
268 cal per serve

250 g frozen mixed berries
1⅓ cups rolled oats

Place the berries in a bowl and defrost in the microwave.

Place the oats and 2⅔ cups of water in a small saucepan. Bring to the boil. Reduce the heat to low and cook for 5 minutes, stirring occasionally.

Divide the oats and serve in two bowls, topping each with half of the berries.

Tip

- For manual workers, adolescents and growing children, increase the calories by serving with ½ cup skim milk (total calories 340) or add 1 tablespoon low-GI sugar to the berries before microwaving (310 calories per serve).

Variations

- Try rhubarb as a topping (see page 188 for poaching instructions; 283 calories per serve) or ½ cup unsweetened stewed apple (274 calories) or pears (286 calories).
- An even easier variation is to stir some fresh berries straight into your porridge (my friends' kids call this 'Purple Porridge').
- For extra energy and sweetness, try adding a small mashed banana (303 calories per serve).

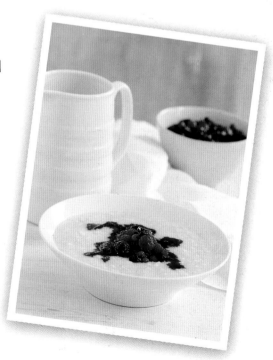

Bran and mixed berries with banana

Serves 2
Prep 5 minutes
340 cal per serve

1 cup processed bran
150 g strawberries,
  hulled and quartered
80 g blueberries
1 banana, sliced
½ cup skim milk

Here's your recommended daily two serves of fruit and you haven't even got out the door yet! The bran is great for the system and the berries and banana will keep you firing all morning.

Divide the bran between 2 bowls. Top with equal serves of the fruit and ¼ cup skim milk.

Fruit and muesli

Serves 2
(Muesli recipe makes 8 serves)
Prep 15 minutes
359 cal per serve

1 small mango, flesh
  cut into cubes
1 kiwi fruit, peeled,
  halved and sliced
1 small banana, sliced
½ cup low-cal plain yoghurt

muesli
2 cups rolled oats
⅔ cup bran
⅓ cup sunflower seeds
⅓ cup pumpkin seeds
¼ cup dried cranberries
¼ cup currants

What a way to start the day! I *always* make my own muesli, because that way I know exactly what's in it. I usually serve it with a little chopped fruit, but sometimes I like to flip the equation and have mostly fruit with just a sprinkling of muesli – it's a great way to bump up my fresh fruit intake while still enjoying the muesli's nutritional benefits. Note that the muesli recipe makes 8 serves (½ cup is one serve), so you can put the rest away for other days.

To make the muesli, combine all the ingredients. Divide 1 cup muesli between 2 bowls. Serve with the fruit and yoghurt. Store the remaining muesli in an airtight container.

Variation

• To make Bircher muesli, combine ½ cup muesli and ½ cup skim milk in a bowl and soak overnight in the fridge. Serve with fresh fruit the next morning.

Bran and mixed berries with banana

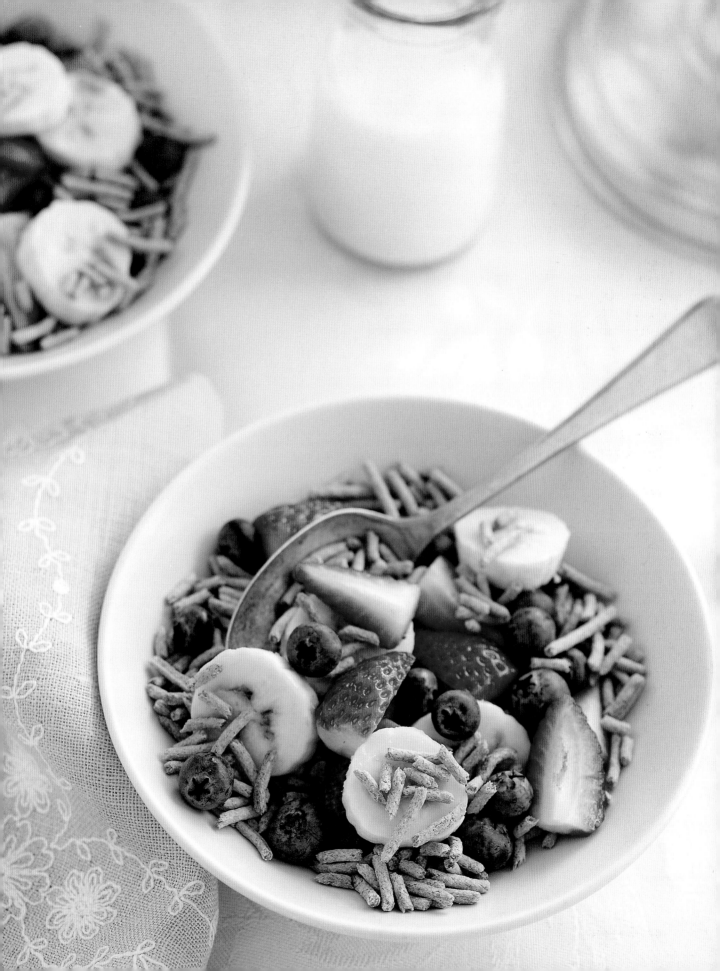

Cottage cheese toast with tomato and rocket

Serves 2
Prep 10 minutes
283 cal per serve

---

250 g low-cal cottage cheese
2 tablespoons finely chopped
  chives
freshly ground black pepper
4 slices wholegrain bread
2 tomatoes, sliced
1 small handful baby rocket

This is definitely the breakfast to impress friends – it ticks all the health boxes, looks amazing and tastes divine. Plus, I love that I am already getting some greens into my diet and it's not even 9 a.m.!

Combine the cottage cheese and chives in a bowl and season to taste with pepper. Toast the bread and spread with the cheese mixture. Top with the tomato and rocket. Season with pepper.

Variations

• Try adding a different herb to the cottage cheese, such as parsley, or add some alfalfa sprouts.
A squeeze of lemon can give a fresh burst as well.
• You could also try this with low-cal ricotta and basil instead of the cottage cheese and chives.
• This is delicious with some smoked salmon. Divide 100 g of salmon between the four slices of toast (place on top of the cheese). Calories will be bumped up to 350 per serve.

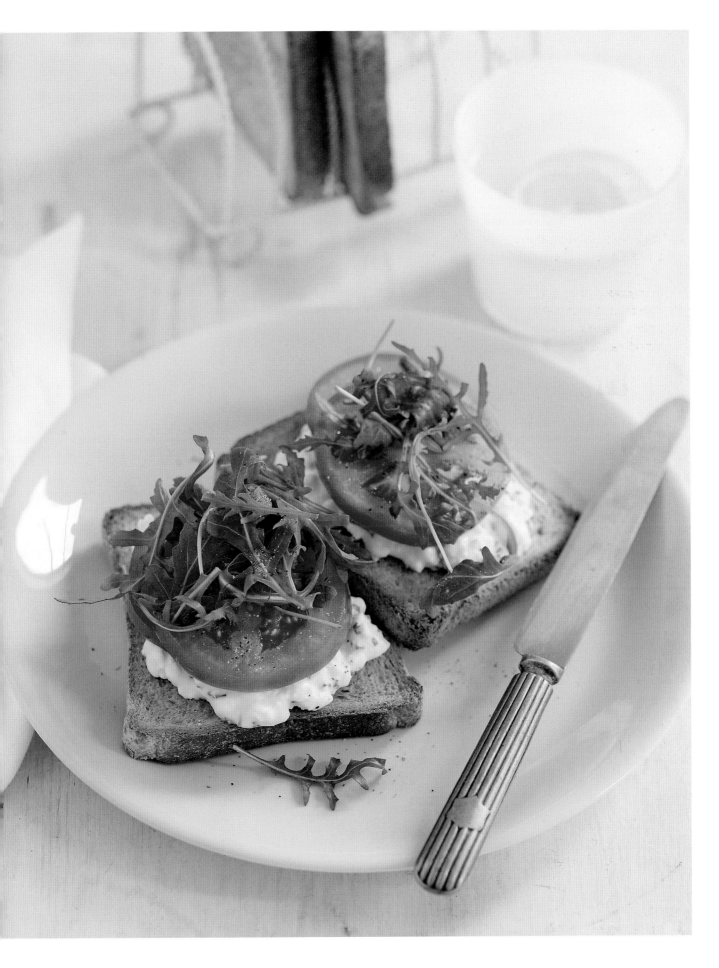

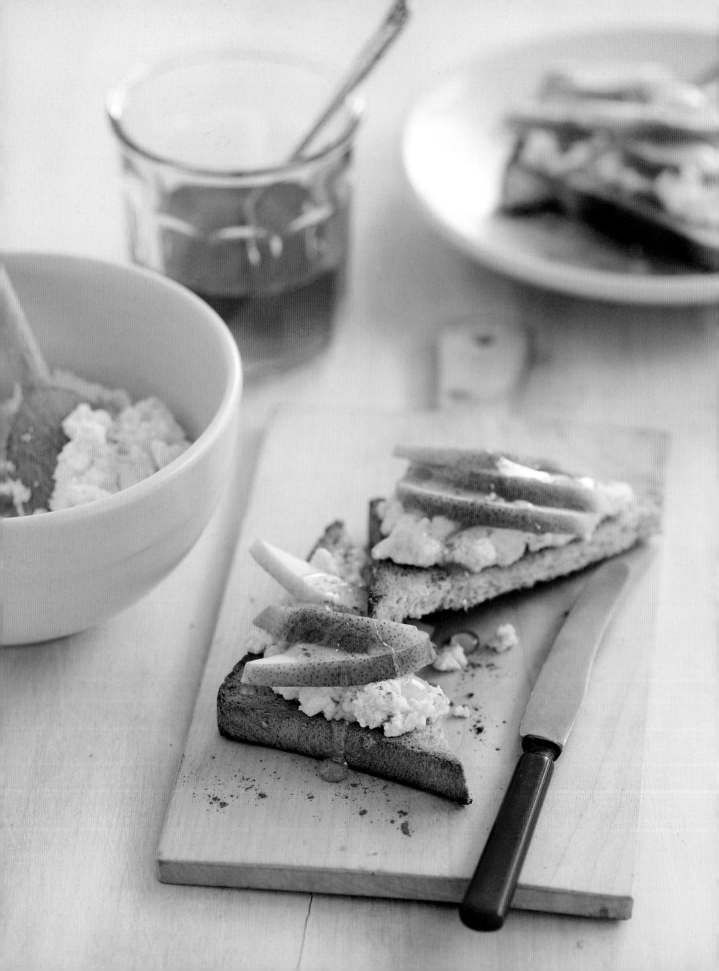

Spiced pear and ricotta toast

This delicious brekkie takes 5 minutes to prepare – that's less time than it takes to make a pot of tea. If it's a chilly morning, warm up the ricotta mix for a few seconds in the microwave – it will help to melt the honey.

Toast the bread. Meanwhile, combine the ricotta, honey and ginger in a bowl. Spread the ricotta mixture over the toast and top with pear slices. Sprinkle with cinnamon to serve.

Tip
- Use a little freshly grated ginger instead of ground ginger for extra zing.

Serves 2
Prep 5 minutes
353 cal per serve

4 slices wholegrain bread
200 g low-cal ricotta
2 teaspoons honey
¼ teaspoon ground ginger
1 pear, cored and sliced
ground cinnamon

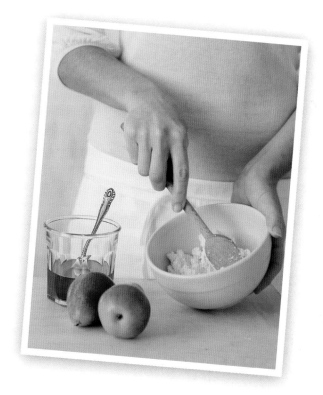

Whole-egg omelette with corn, spinach and dill

Serves 2
Prep 10 minutes
Cook 5 minutes
389 cal per serve

1 large corn cob, leaves removed
2 large eggs
40 g low-cal feta, crumbled
1 shallot, thinly sliced
2 teaspoons finely chopped fresh
   dill, plus extra fronds to garnish
freshly ground black pepper
4 slices wholegrain bread
olive oil spray
50 g cherry tomatoes, halved
1 large handful baby spinach
   leaves

This is another terrific breakfast I make on weekends (I've even had this for dinner minus the bread). As you can see it's easy to prepare. It's also a dish where I can vary the vegetables to get a completely new flavour sensation. I tend to steer clear of vegies with a high water content (which can make the omelette slushy) and go for tangy options like garlic chives or shallots.

Cut the corn from the cob and cook in a small saucepan of boiling water for 5 minutes until tender. Drain.

Break the eggs into a bowl and lightly beat with a fork until just combined. Stir in the corn, feta, shallot and chopped dill. Season with pepper.

Toast the bread. Meanwhile, lightly spray a medium non-stick frying pan with olive oil and heat on medium–high. Add half the egg mixture. Cook for 2 minutes until just set. Top with half the tomatoes and half the spinach. Fold over and slide onto a warm plate, or serve open in a shallow bowl topped with the tomatoes and spinach. Keep warm. Repeat with the remaining egg mixture, tomatoes and spinach.

Garnish the omelettes with dill fronds, and serve with the toast.

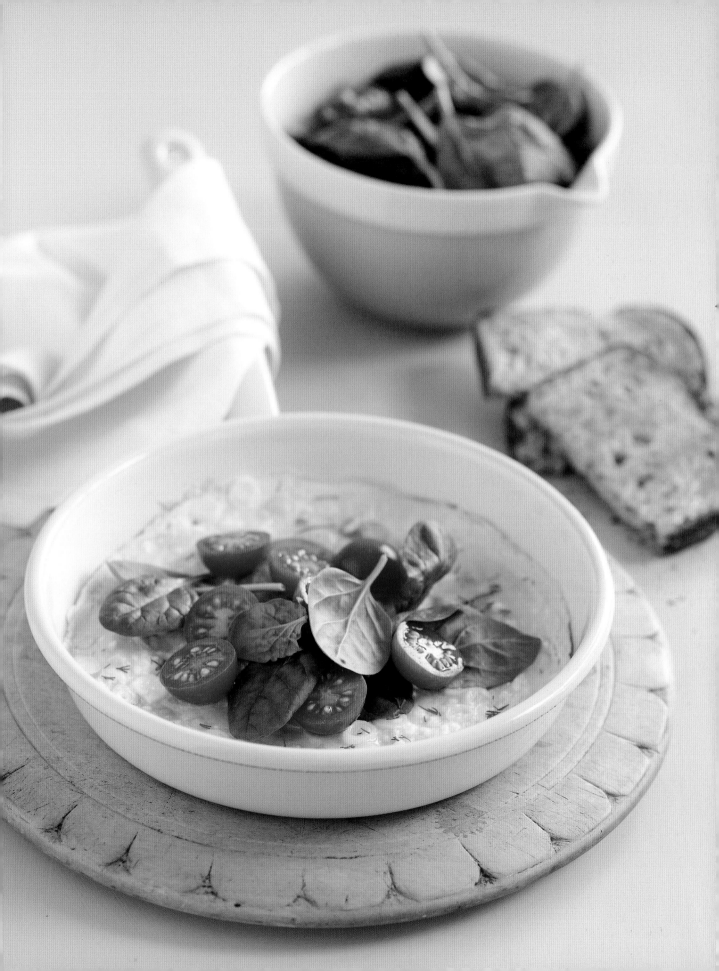

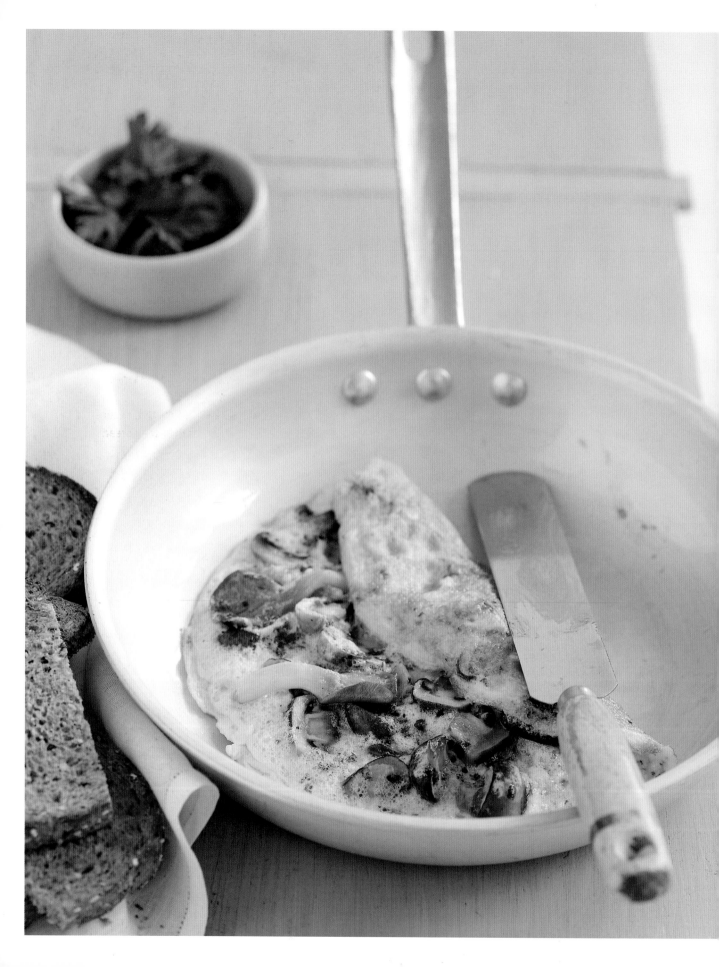

Egg-white omelette
with garlic mushrooms

Nothing, but nothing, beats this high-protein, low-calorie breakfast.
I especially love it after training – the garlic mushrooms are to die for.
Some people leave one egg yolk in the mix, but if you do you'll need to
add 50–70 calories (depending on the size of the egg) to your daily count.

Serves 2
Prep 10 minutes
Cook 10 minutes
300 cal per serve

Lightly spray a frying pan with oil and heat on medium–high.
Cook the mushrooms for 6 minutes, stirring, until browned.
Stir in the garlic, parsley and shallot and cook for 30 seconds
until fragrant. Remove from the heat.

Whisk the egg whites in a bowl until combined. Stir through
the mushroom mixture and season to taste with pepper.

Toast the bread. Meanwhile, lightly spray a medium non-stick
frying pan with olive oil and heat on medium–high. Pour in half
of the egg-white mixture and cook for 1–2 minutes until just set.
Fold over and slide onto a warm plate. Keep warm. Repeat with
the remaining egg-white mixture for the second omelette.

Serve the omelettes with the toast.

olive oil spray
250 g mixed fresh mushrooms
   (oyster, Swiss brown, shimeji),
   sliced
1 garlic clove, crushed
2 tablespoons freshly chopped
   parsley
1 shallot, finely chopped
10 egg whites
freshly ground black pepper
4 slices wholegrain bread

Beans on toast with fried egg

Serves 2
(Bean mix serves 4)
Prep 5 minutes
Cook 15 minutes
360 cal per serve

---

2 medium eggs
4 slices wholegrain bread
1 tablespoon freshly chopped
    parsley

bean mix
olive oil spray
1 onion, finely chopped
1 garlic clove, crushed
2 × 400 g cans cannellini beans,
    drained and rinsed
400 g can diced tomatoes
1½ teaspoons mustard powder
1 teaspoon Worcestershire sauce
freshly ground black pepper

This is a total winner for weekend breakfasts and just lovely during winter. The beans are low-GI carbohydrates, so you will be full all morning and still have plenty of energy for that afternoon touch-football game in the park with your mates and kids. Try making up more of the bean mix and freezing it in individual portions for later.

To make the beans (about 2⅓ cups or 4 single serves), lightly spray a saucepan with olive oil and heat on medium. Cook the onion and garlic, stirring, for 5 minutes until softened but not coloured. Add the beans, tomatoes, mustard powder and Worcestershire sauce. Simmer for 8 minutes, stirring occasionally, until the beans are very soft and the sauce has thickened. Season to taste with pepper.

Lightly spray a non-stick frying pan with olive oil and heat on medium–high. Break the eggs into the pan and cook for 1–2 minutes until the whites are set. Slide onto 2 warm plates.

Toast the bread. For each person, top 1 slice of toast with about ½ cup hot beans, sprinkle with parsley and serve with another slice of toast.

Tips

• Store leftover bean mix in an airtight container in the fridge. The bean mix is 580 calories all up (to serve 4).

• I prefer to use dried beans rather than canned ones because they taste better. Follow the directions on the pack for soaking and/or boiling 1 cup dried beans and use as described above.

• I often have some leftover beans on 2 slices of toast for lunch the next day – without the egg. Just heat ½ cup of bean mix in the microwave and serve on toast (265 calories).

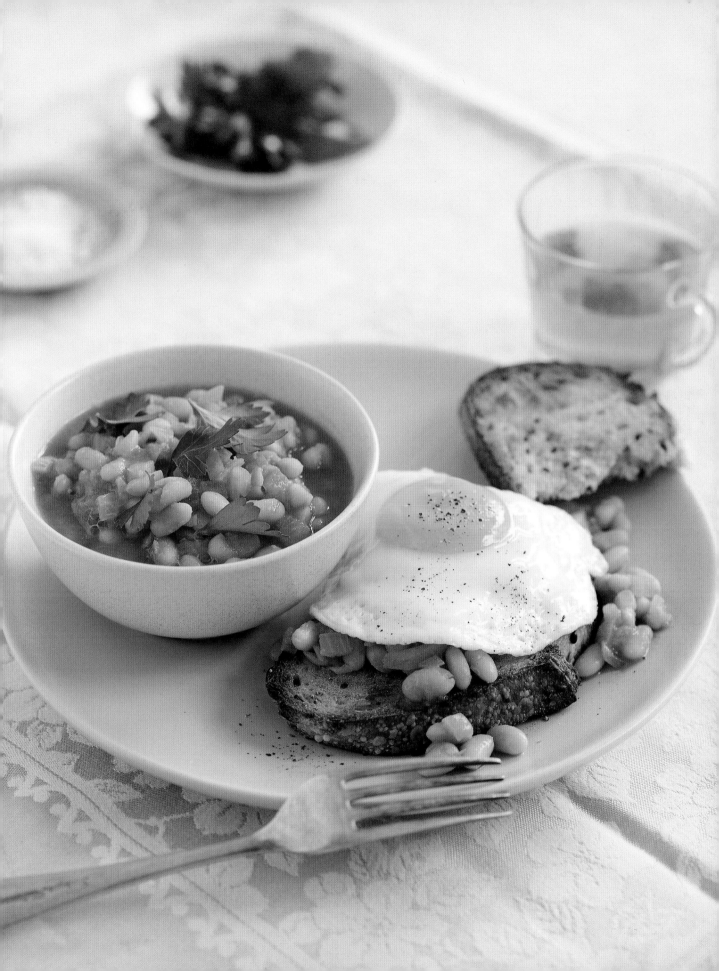

Scrambled eggs with grilled asparagus and tomatoes

Serves 2
Prep 5 minutes
Cook 10 minutes
335 cal per serve

olive oil spray
1 bunch asparagus, trimmed
150 g cherry tomatoes
   (preferably truss)
2 large eggs, lightly beaten
¼ cup low-cal ricotta
4 slices wholegrain bread
freshly ground black pepper
2 tablespoons baby basil leaves

Now these scrambled eggs are my style – totally yummy, but without the calories. The grilled vegies are just so tasty, and of course getting extra vegetables into your diet is fantastic.

Lightly spray a char-grill pan with olive oil and heat on medium–high. Grill the asparagus for 4 minutes. Add the tomatoes and cook for another 4 minutes until the asparagus and tomatoes are lightly charred.

Meanwhile, lightly spray a non-stick saucepan or frying pan with olive oil and heat on high. Add the eggs and cook, stirring, for 1–2 minutes until starting to set. Remove from the heat and stir in the ricotta.

Toast the bread, then spoon the egg mixture onto the toast (2 slices per serve). Season with pepper and garnish with basil. Serve with the grilled tomatoes and asparagus.

Variation

* If you don't have any fresh basil handy, sprinkle in some dried herbs instead, or better yet add finely chopped shallots or fresh parsley.

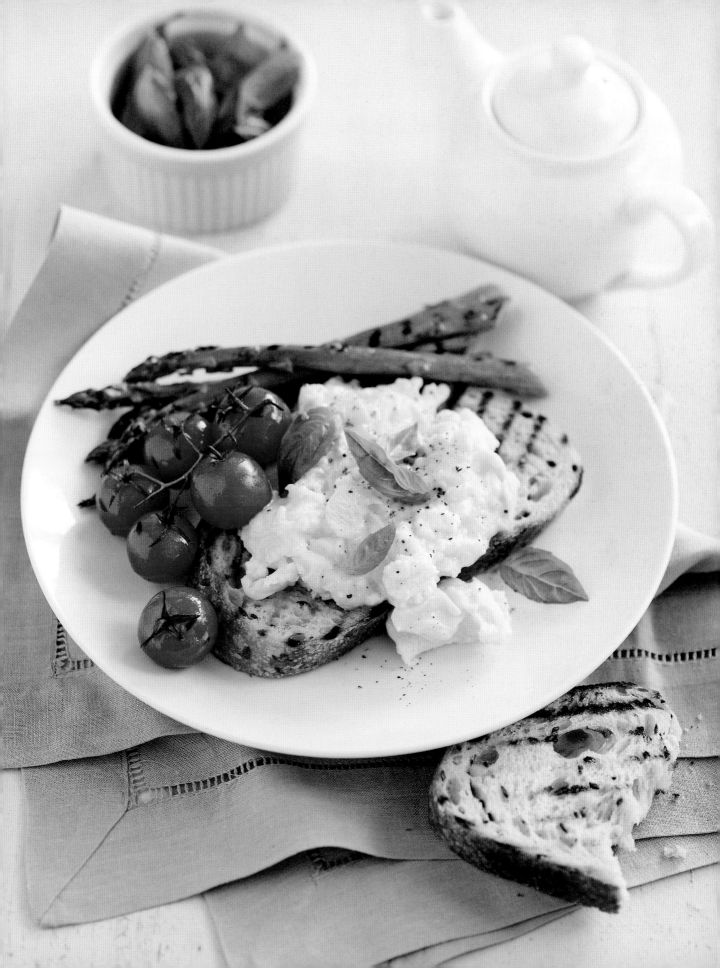

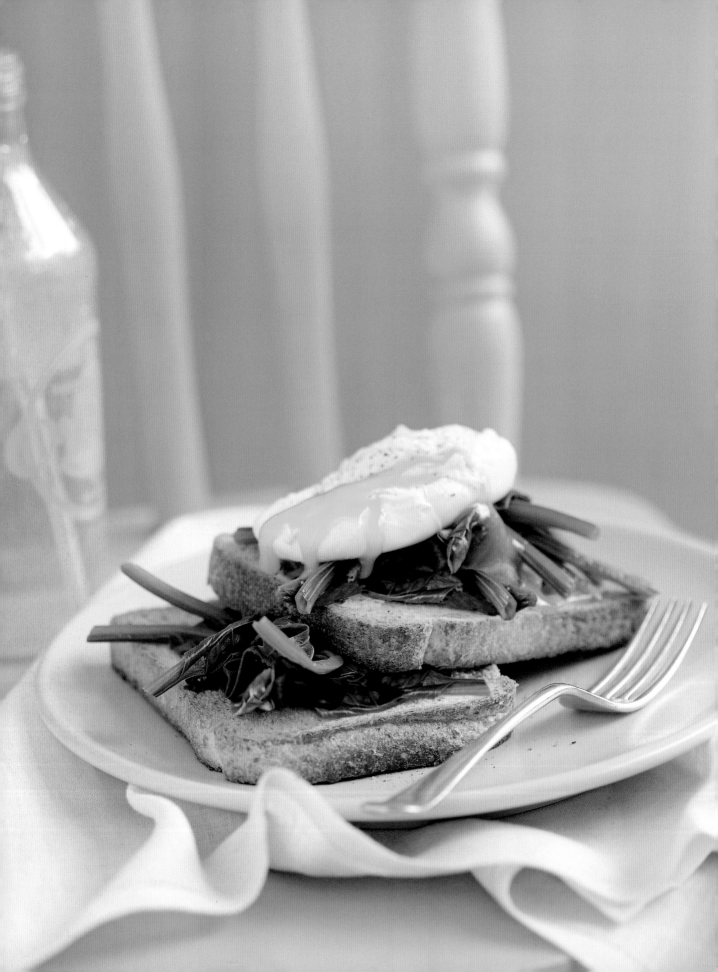

Poached eggs on garlic toast with wilted spinach

Eggs are an amazing breakfast food, but the calories can quickly get out of hand if the eggs are fried, or are scrambled with a couple of dollops of cream. Poached is always the best way to go, and in this recipe, I'm also getting some greens into my diet right at the start of the day.

Serves 2
Prep 10 minutes
Cook 5 minutes
290 cal per serve

olive oil spray
1 bunch spinach, well washed and trimmed
1 teaspoon white vinegar
2 large eggs
4 slices wholemeal or soy-and-linseed bread
1 garlic clove
freshly ground black pepper

Lightly spray a large non-stick frying pan with olive oil and heat on high. Add the spinach and stir-fry for 2 minutes until just wilted. Season to taste with pepper and keep warm.

Half-fill a small saucepan with water and add the vinegar. Bring almost to the boil and, just as the little bubbles are rising to the surface, reduce the heat a bit and stir the water vigorously to create a whirlpool (don't scald yourself). Carefully crack 1 egg on the side of the saucepan and release the contents into the middle of the whirlpool – this will stop the white going all over the place. Fish the poached egg out with a slotted spoon after 2 minutes for a softie, or 3 minutes for a hardie. Repeat with the other egg.

Toast the bread, then rub 2 slices of toast with the garlic. Top each slice with spinach and a poached egg. Season with pepper and serve with the remaining toast.

Tips
● Wash the spinach well, as soil often gets trapped in the inner leaves.
● The vinegar helps to set the protein in the egg so that it holds its shape. If you don't like the taste of vinegar, rinse the egg under hot water after poaching.

Variations
● Top your toast with a small thinly sliced zucchini (301 calories per serve).
● Divide 100 g smoked salmon between your toast slices (350 calories per serve).

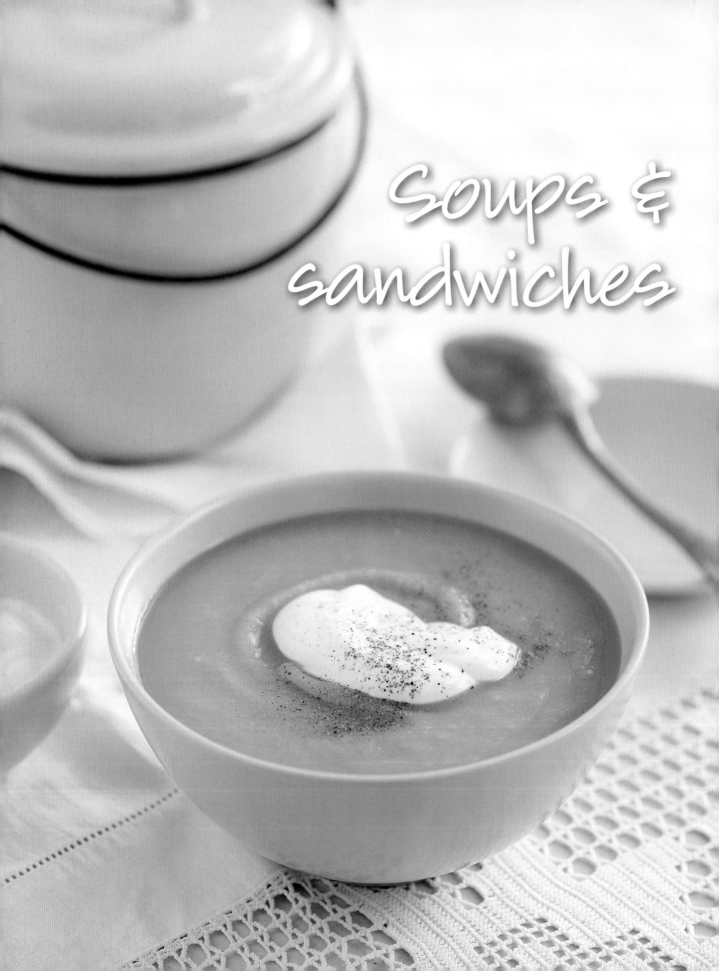

Soups & sandwiches

Pumpkin soup

Pumpkin soup doesn't have to be as big on the calories as you might expect.
This recipe is especially delicious if you use freshly ground cumin seeds.
I've got a Jamie Oliver Flavour Shaker, and it's great for crushing seeds and
spices in small quantities. The aroma is amazing!

Heat the oil in a large saucepan on medium. Cook the onion and
garlic stirring for 5 minutes, until soft and transparent (not coloured).
Stir in the pumpkin and cumin and cook for another minute until
fragrant. Add the chicken stock and 2 cups of water. Bring to the boil
and simmer, covered, for 15 minutes, until the pumpkin is tender.

Cool slightly and puree in batches, using a food processor or hand-
held blender. Season with pepper to taste.

Serve with a dollop of yoghurt and garnish with coriander.

Tips
- This soup makes 8 cups – 2 cups per serve.
- I've made the soup quite thick. If you prefer it thinner,
just add another cup of water when cooking.
- This soup also freezes well. Remember to label and
date your containers.

Serves 4
Prep 10 minutes
Cook 20 minutes
227 cal per serve

1 tablespoon olive oil
1 onion, chopped
2 garlic cloves, chopped
1.8 kg butternut pumpkin,
    seeded, cut into chunks
½ teaspoon cumin seeds
2 cups (500 ml) salt-reduced
    chicken stock
freshly ground black pepper
⅓ cup plain low-cal yoghurt
coriander sprigs, to garnish

Minestrone

Serves 4
Prep 10 minutes
Cook 20 minutes
294 cal per serve

1 tablespoon olive oil
1 onion, chopped
2 garlic cloves, crushed
4 cups vegetable stock
2 tablespoons salt-reduced
   tomato paste
1 large carrot, diced
1 celery stick, diced
1 cup dried macaroni
400 g tin butter beans,
   drained, rinsed
300 g cabbage, coarsely shredded
1 zucchini, diced
freshly ground black pepper
2 tablespoons freshly torn basil
2 tablespoons shaved parmesan

Classic minestrone is a delicious, filling vegetarian dish – just perfect on a cold day. This recipe makes 10 cups (enough for 4–5 serves), so freeze your leftovers or pop them in the fridge for another meal.

Heat the oil in a large saucepan on medium. Cook the onion and garlic for 5 minutes, stirring until softened. Add the stock, tomato paste and 2 cups of water and stir until combined. Add the carrot, celery, macaroni and beans. Gently boil for 5 minutes. Add the cabbage and zucchini and gently boil for another 8 minutes until the vegetables are tender and the pasta is cooked.

To serve, season with pepper and garnish with basil and parmesan.

Tip

- If you don't have any fresh basil, use 1 teaspoon dried basil.

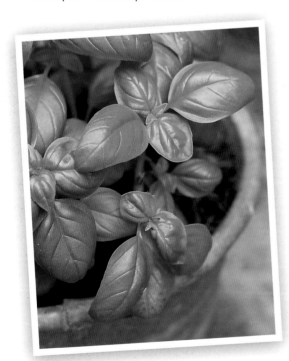

Leek and asparagus soup

Leeks are like onions, but with a more delicate flavour. This delicious variation of leek and potato soup makes about 8 cups, is super-low in calories and is a good one for the freezer.

Cut asparagus into 4 cm lengths and separate tips and stalks. Cook tips in boiling, salted water for 1 minute. Drain and refresh under cold water. Halve tips and set aside.

Heat the oil in a large saucepan on medium. Stir in the asparagus stalks, leek and potato. Cook, covered, for 10 minutes stirring occasionally until soft without colouring. Add stock and 3 cups of water. Bring to the boil and simmer covered for 8–10 minutes.

Puree soup in batches, using a blender or food processor. Reheat and season to taste. Serve garnished with asparagus tips and chives.

Serves 4
Prep 10 minutes
Cook 20 minutes
162 cal per serve

3 bunches asparagus, trimmed
1 tablespoon olive oil
2 leeks, washed, sliced,
   with 5 cm of green left on
1 large potato, diced
3 cups salt-reduced chicken stock
½ bunch chives, finely chopped

Tips

- If you don't have a food processor, it's worth investing in a hand-held blender. They're inexpensive and easy to store and usually come with a small attachment for chopping herbs.
- Asparagus stalks can be woody. To trim, hold asparagus spears in the middle and snap off the ends.
- Leeks have layered leaves which make them tricky to clean. Cut off the root base and make a cut along the centre of the leek almost to the cut end but not quite, so the leaves stay together. Then rinse it under the tap fanning out the leaves as you do so.
- Bring the soup to room temperature before freezing in airtight containers. Thaw and reheat in a microwave, or in a saucepan on medium heat.

Variation

- Chop a sprig of mint and use instead of the chives. Yum!

Beef and ramen noodle soup

Serves 2
Prep 15 minutes
Cook 10 minutes
351 cal per serve

3 cups salt-reduced beef stock
3 teaspoons fish sauce
1 tablespoon salt-reduced
   soy sauce
4 cm piece ginger, peeled
2 star anise
2 cinnamon sticks
100 g dried ramen noodles
100 g bean sprouts
160 g rump steak, trimmed
   and sliced paper-thin
2 shallots, sliced thinly on
   the diagonal
½ cup freshly chopped coriander
1 lime, juice only, plus extra lime
   wedges to serve

Here's another hearty, inexpensive tastebud pleaser. Make sure you use proper dried ramen noodles, not the ones that come prepackaged in Styrofoam cups.

Place the stock, fish sauce, soy sauce, ginger, star anise, cinnamon sticks and 3 cups water in a saucepan. Bring to the boil and simmer for 5 minutes. Remove the ginger, star anise and cinnamon sticks with a slotted spoon and discard.

Meanwhile, cook the ramen noodles according to the packet directions. Drain and place in 2 serving bowls. Top with the bean sprouts, beef slices, shallots and coriander.

Reheat the stock until almost boiling, then stir in the lime juice. Ladle the hot stock over the noodles and beef. Serve immediately with lime wedges on the side.

Tips

• To get paper-thin beef slices, place the beef in the freezer for 1 hour before slicing.
• Make a double or triple batch of the stock and freeze for another time. Increase the quantity of the liquids accordingly, but use the same amounts of ginger and spices.

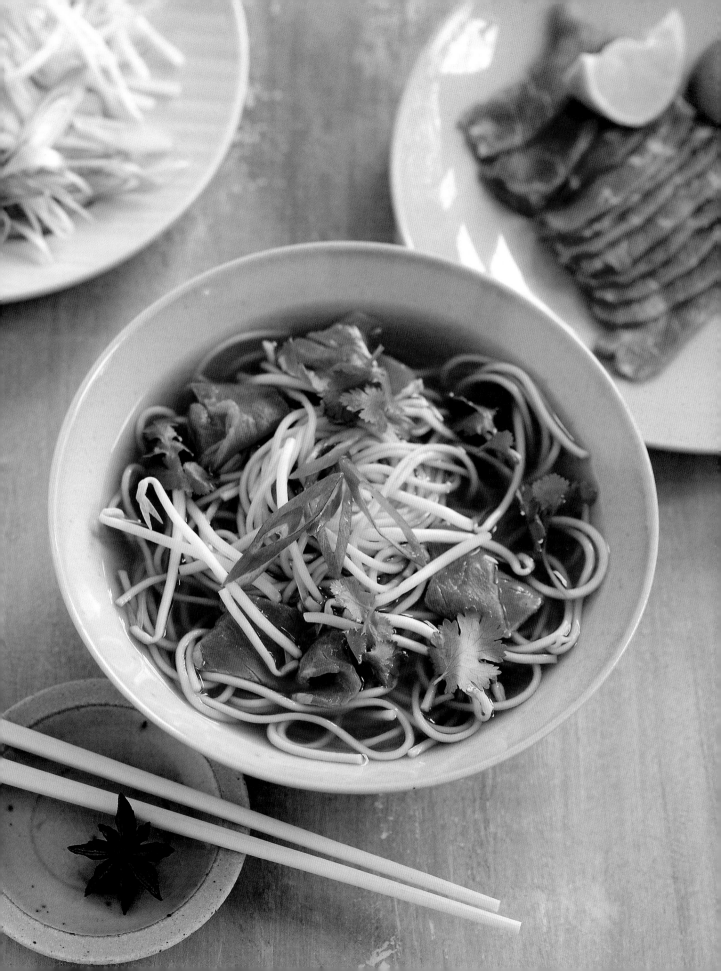

Chicken and vegetable soup with silverbeet

Serves 2
(Vegetable soup base serves 6)
Prep 15 minutes
Cook 20 minutes
317 cal per serve

220 g skinless chicken thigh
  fillets, trimmed and cut into
  bite-sized pieces
100 g silverbeet leaves, washed
  and finely shredded

vegetable soup base
1 onion, chopped
2 garlic cloves, crushed
3 anchovies, drained and
  finely chopped (optional)
1 litre (about 4 cups)
  salt-reduced chicken stock
3 large carrots, halved
  lengthways and sliced
3 large celery sticks, sliced
3 medium turnips, peeled,
  quartered and sliced
150 g green beans, trimmed
  and halved
400 g can borlotti beans,
  drained and rinsed

This is an important recipe to learn, as the vegetable soup base can be used for a variety of other meals. You'll notice that the quantities I've used allow for plenty of soup for future use (the soup base makes about 12 cups, which is about 6 serves).

To make the vegetable soup base, lightly spray a large saucepan with oil and heat on medium. Cook the onion, garlic and anchovy (if using) for 5 minutes, stirring, until the onion softens. Add the stock and 5 cups water. Bring to the boil, then add the remaining vegetables. Simmer, covered, for 10 minutes until the vegetables are tender. Ladle 4 serves into individual containers and freeze or refrigerate for another use.

Bring the remaining 2 serves to the boil. Stir in the chicken and silverbeet and simmer gently for 2 minutes until the chicken is cooked through and the silverbeet is bright green. Serve immediately.

Tip

- Chicken thighs are cheaper than chicken breasts, but they are fattier – so be sure to take off all the skin and trim them carefully.

Tom yum soup with rice crackers

Tom yum is a versatile, low-calorie clear soup – you can add chicken, prawns or even fish. I like my food spicy, so I add extra chilli for a bit more bite. Watch out for the crackers, though – they can be as much as 10 calories each, so don't ruin your low-calorie meal by tucking in to the bikkies!

Place 4 cups of water in a saucepan and bring to the boil. Stir in the tom yum paste until combined. Add the corn and simmer for 5 minutes. Add the mushrooms and simmer for another 5 minutes. Stir in the soy sauce and baby bok choy.

Garnish soup with coriander and shallot and serve with lime wedges and crackers.

Variations

- For even more flavour, use chicken broth left over from the Chinese poached chicken (page 161) instead of water.
- This is also delicious with 200 g sliced chicken breast (264 calories per serve) or 200 g peeled green prawns (218 calories per serve). Simply add the chicken or prawns along with the mushrooms and simmer for 5 minutes until cooked through.

Serves 2
Prep 10 minutes
Cook 10 minutes
129 cal per serve

2 teaspoons tom yum paste
60 g baby corn, halved on the diagonal
50 g shiitake mushrooms, sliced
2 teaspoons salt-reduced soy sauce
1 bunch baby bok choy, leaves separated
1 cup coriander leaves
1 shallot, sliced on the diagonal
1 lime, cut into wedges, to serve
12 plain Sakata rice crackers

Chicken and avocado sandwich

Serves 2
Prep 5 minutes
300 cal per sandwich

4 slices wholemeal bread
¼ small avocado
70 g cooked lean chicken,
    shredded
½ small celery stick, thinly sliced
1 tablespoon freshly chopped
    parsley
1 shallot bulb, thinly sliced
1 handful snowpea sprouts
freshly ground black pepper

This is my favourite chicken sandwich mix. Don't get hung up on making sure that you have the exact salad ingredients – you can always tinker with them to suit your palate or what's in your fridge. Keep the avocado to a very, very light smear – avocados are nutritious, but very high in calories. Because I'm adding extra calories with the chicken, I always use less avocado than I do with my salad sandwich.

Spread the bread with the avocado. Top 2 slices of bread with chicken, celery, parsley, shallot and sprouts. Season to taste with pepper and cover with the remaining slices of bread.

Tip
• Use leftover chicken, or cook an extra portion of chicken on the weekend and keep it in the fridge ready for lunches.

Variation
• Instead of avocado use a smear of low-fat mayonnaise or 2 tablespoons of tzatziki (see page 202).

Chicken and avocado sandwich (front);
Chicken, eggplant and hummus sandwich (back)

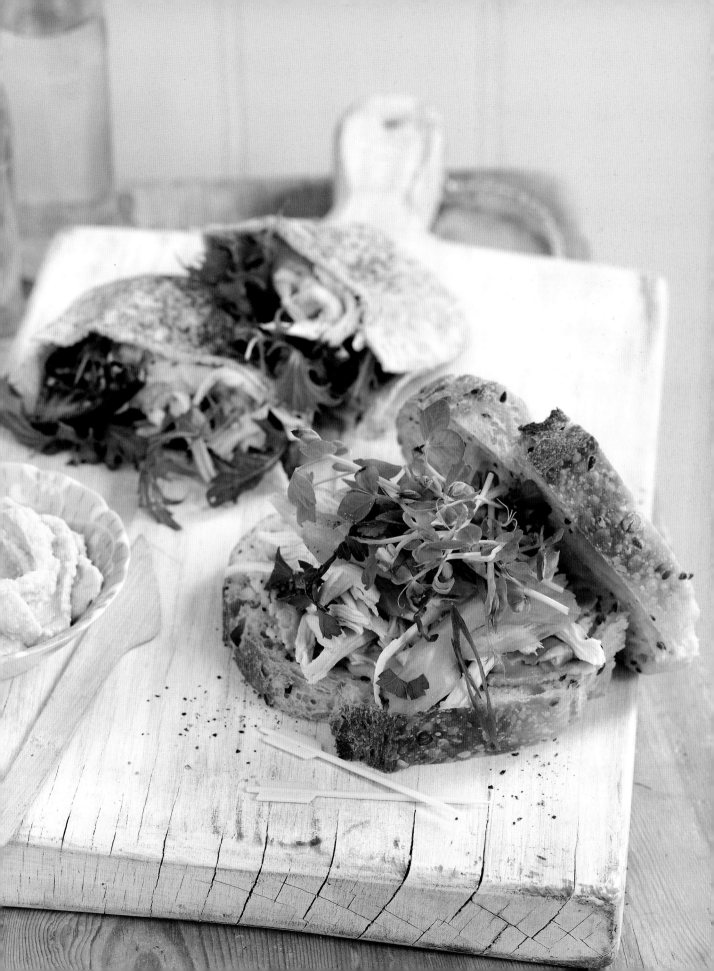

Chicken, eggplant and hummus sandwich

Serves 2
Prep 5 minutes
276 cal per sandwich

50 g eggplant
olive oil spray
2 wholemeal pita pockets
¼ cup hummus (see page 200)
70 g cooked lean chicken,
  shredded
1 handful mixed salad leaves

Pita bread makes a nice change from sliced wholemeal, and the calories are the same. Go easy with the hummus, as it's a high-calorie item – just a light smear.

Cut eggplant into thin slices. Spray lightly with olive oil and cook on a char-grill pan until lightly charred and tender. Drain on paper towel.

Using a small knife, make a slit in each pita to open the pocket. Thinly spread one side of the cavity with hummus and fill with eggplant, chicken and salad leaves.

Tip
● Grill your eggplant the night before and store in the refrigerator in an airtight container.

See page 77 for photograph.

Mediterranean sandwich with olive and basil tapenade

The great thing with tapenade is that although it uses high-calorie ingredients, you don't need a lot of it to really enjoy the flavour. Just a smear is all it takes.

To make the tapenade, puree the olives, anchovies, capers, basil and garlic using a food processor or blender. Stir through the oil and season with pepper.

Spread 2 bread slices with 1 tablespoon tapenade each. Add the artichoke, rocket and grilled capsicum and top with remaining bread.

Tip
- Store tapenade in an airtight container in the fridge for up to 1 month.

Variations
- Try tomato, basil and rocket with the tapenade (166 calories), or tuna, rocket and artichoke (209 calories).
- Chicken, bean sprouts and grilled eggplant is also delicious with tapenade (219 calories).

Serves 2
(Tapenade makes 1¼ cups)
Prep 15 minutes
176 cal per sandwich
31 cal per teaspoon tapenade

4 slices wholemeal or
  seeded bread
3 artichoke hearts, thinly sliced
1 handful rocket
100 g grilled capsicum
  (see page 106)

olive and basil tapenade
2 cups black olives, pitted and
  rinsed
2 anchovy fillets
2 tablespoons capers, rinsed
1 cup basil leaves
1 garlic clove, crushed
1 tablespoon extra virgin olive oil
freshly ground black pepper

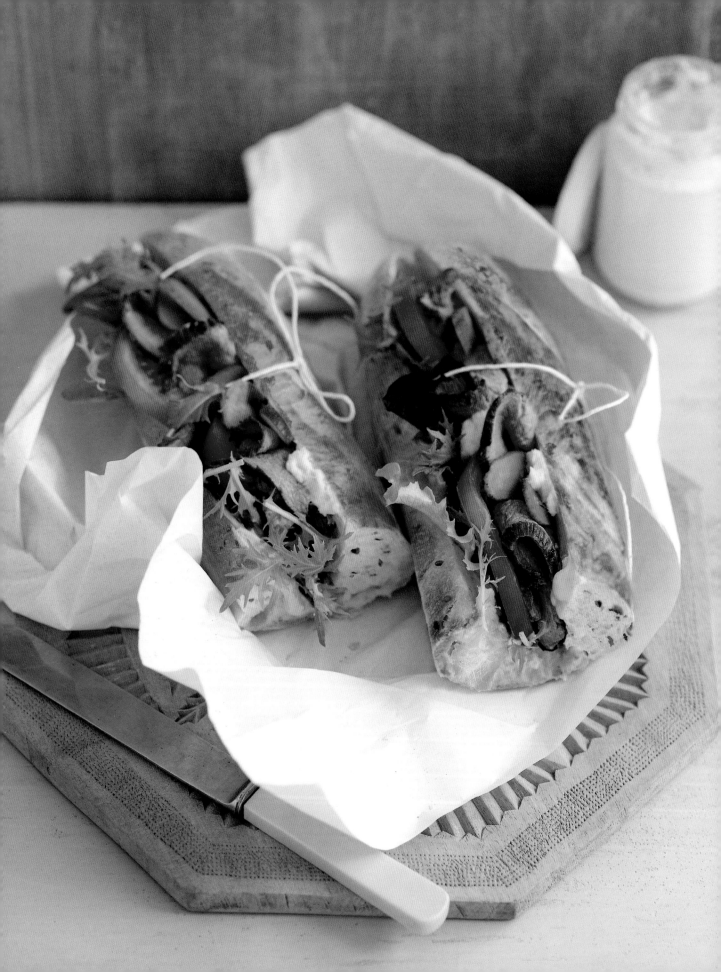

Roast beef sandwich

Here's where I use some of the delicious roast beef I've cooked for my mum on the weekend (see page 181). You could also use some beef from my Thai beef salad (page 104) if you cook a little extra. The key to a good roast beef sanger is to slice the beef thinly, so keep your knives sharp and take your time.

Using a serrated knife, split the bread open. Spread the base with mustard and top with horseradish. Fill with the mixed leaves, tomato, roast beef and gherkins.

Variation

● Use whatever salad filling you have in the fridge: e.g. if you don't have gherkins, try olives.

Serves 2
Prep 5 minutes
317 cal per sandwich

½ breadstick, halved widthways
1 tablespoon Dijon mustard
1 teaspoon horseradish
1 handful mixed salad leaves
1 tomato, sliced
80 g very thinly sliced roast beef
2 large gherkins, sliced
  lengthways

Mixed herb, ricotta and tomato wrap

This great, fresh-tasting wrap really fills you up. Chives and parsley are easily grown in the garden, so if you're a bit of a gardener you can enjoy this lunchtime meal with the freshest of produce!

Combine the ricotta, herbs and garlic in a small bowl. Spread over the bread. Place the mixed leaves, tomato and celery at one end of the bread, then roll tightly to enclose the filling. Halve each wrap using a sharp knife.

Variation

● If you're short of time, try filling the bread with some leftover coleslaw (see page 100) or the chicken with fennel, cabbage, radish and cranberry coleslaw (see page 94). Half a cup is 46 calories.

Serves 2
Prep 15 minutes
214 cal per wrap

200 g low-cal ricotta
½ cup chopped chives and parsley
  or other mixed fresh herbs
½ garlic clove, crushed
2 slices mountain bread
2 handfuls mixed salad leaves
1 tomato, sliced
1 small celery stick, finely sliced

Smoked salmon and avocado wrap with watercress

Serves 2
Prep 5 minutes
318 cal per wrap

½ small avocado, mashed
2 slices mountain bread
120 g smoked salmon
2 handfuls watercress
½ Lebanese cucumber,
  thinly sliced
⅛ small red onion, thinly sliced

What I love most about this recipe is the watercress. It's a lovely peppery herb that brings the whole wrap to life. Go very easy with the avocado – it can be lethal when it comes to calories. Use a shallot if you don't have a red onion.

Spread the avocado thinly over the bread. Place some salmon, watercress, cucumber and onion at one end and roll tightly to enclose the filling. Halve each roll with a sharp knife.

Salad sandwich

Serves 2
Prep 10 minutes
310 cal per sandwich

4 slices wholemeal or
  seeded bread
½ small avocado, mashed
freshly ground black pepper
½ Lebanese cucumber, sliced
½ cup alfalfa sprouts
½ carrot, grated
50 g canned sliced beetroot,
  drained
½ tomato, sliced

A summer staple. Go easy with the avocado – just a smear. Sometimes I leave out the avocado and use low-fat mayo or cottage cheese instead. I haven't included onions in this recipe, but if you like an onion flavour, chop up some shallots and scatter them over the other ingredients.

Spread 2 bread slices thinly with the avocado and season to taste with pepper. Add the remaining ingredients and top with the other 2 slices of bread.

Variations
● Try this with 3 tablespoons tzatziki (see page 202) or hummus (page 200) instead of avocado (both 290 calories).

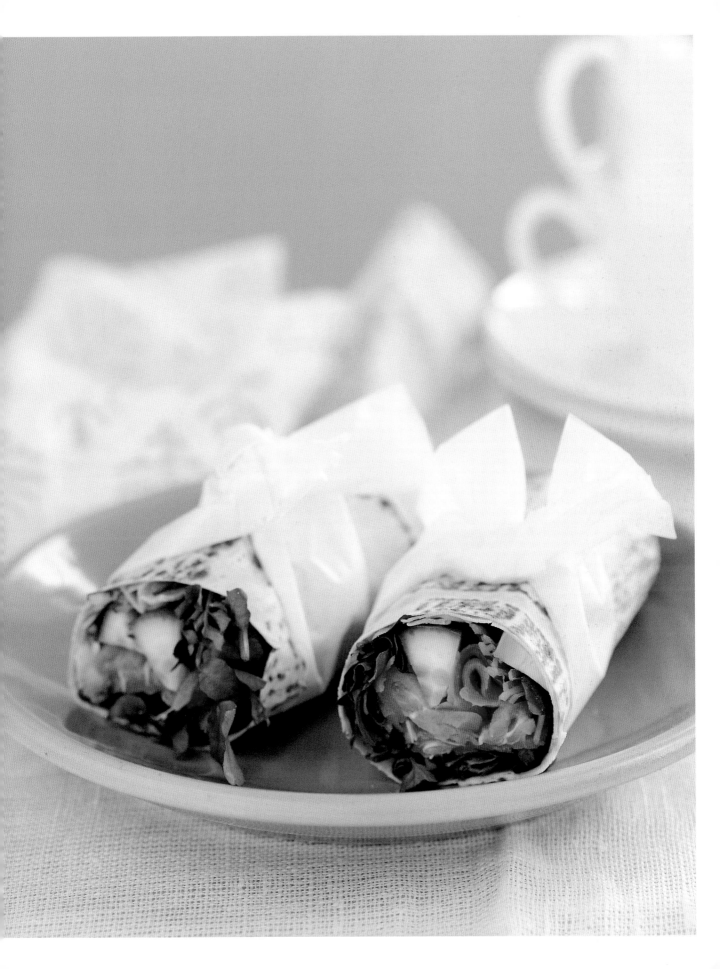

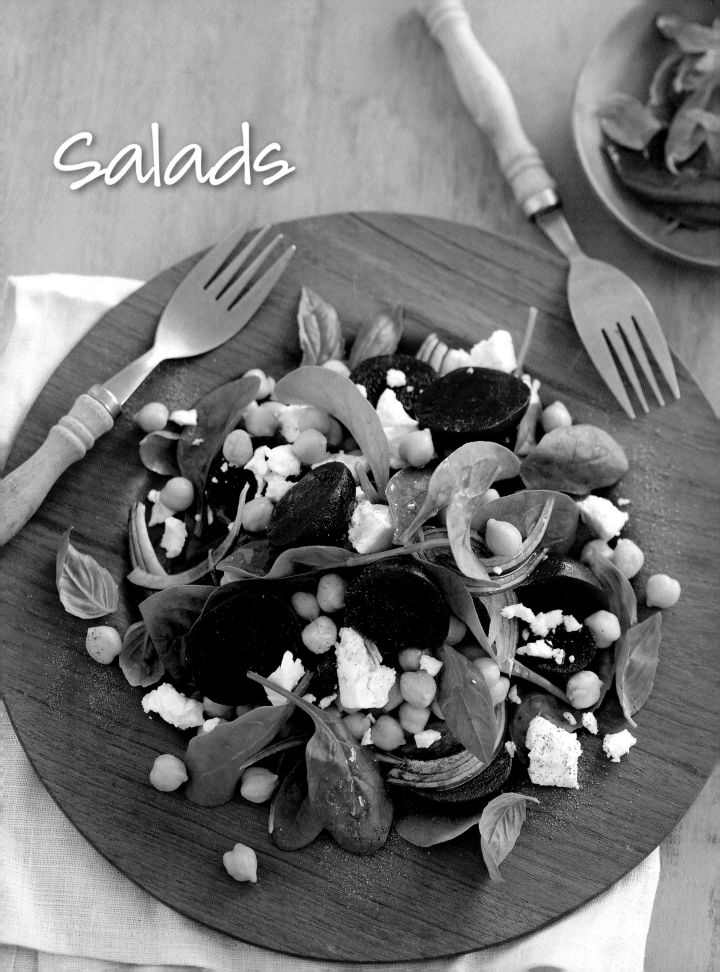

Salads

Baby beet, chickpea, basil and feta salad

A salad that gets full marks for presentation! I love the colours – the purple beetroot, the green basil, the golden chickpeas, topped off with snow-white feta. If canned beetroot is too tart for your taste, try cooking your own (see page 168).

Combine baby beets, chickpeas, baby spinach, red onion and basil in a salad bowl. Drizzle over combined oil and vinegar. Season with freshly ground black pepper and toss to coat. Crumble over feta.

Variation

● Try this salad with 300 g roasted pumpkin instead of beetroot. Place chunks, slices or wedges of pumpkin on a baking tray. Lightly spray with oil and roast for 30-40 minutes (depending on thickness) in a 220°C oven.

Serves 2
Prep 10 minutes
327 cal per serve

440 g can whole baby beets, drained
400 g can chickpeas, drained, rinsed
4 handfuls baby spinach
¼ red onion, thinly sliced
2 tablespoon freshly torn basil
1 tablespoon extra virgin olive oil
1 tablespoon white balsamic vinegar
freshly ground black pepper
40 g low-cal feta

Buckwheat noodle salad with sesame seeds

Serves 2
Prep 15 minutes
Cook 10 minutes
353 cal per serve

1 tablespoon mirin
3 teaspoons rice wine vinegar
2 teaspoons soy sauce
1 garlic clove, crushed
1 bunch asparagus, trimmed
150 g dried buckwheat soba
   noodles
1 small red capsicum, thinly sliced
1 Lebanese cucumber, halved
   lengthways, cut into thin strips
½ cup chopped coriander
1 teaspoon sesame oil
freshly ground black pepper
2 teaspoons sesame seeds,
   roasted

Who would ever have imagined a noodle salad could taste this good? Mirin is like a sugary sake (rice wine) and gives this dish a distinctive sweet flavour. This salad is a real crowd pleaser.

To make the dressing, combine mirin, vinegar, soy sauce and garlic in a small bowl.

Cook the asparagus in a saucepan of boiling, salted water for 2 minutes. Remove with a slotted spoon and cool under cold water. Cut the asparagus heads from the stems and halve lengthways. Cut the stems into thin 6 cm strips.

Cook the noodles in the asparagus water according to the packet directions. Drain and rinse under cold water. Drain again. Transfer to a salad bowl with asparagus, capsicum, cucumber, coriander and sesame oil. Add dressing and toss to coat. Season with pepper and sprinkle with sesame seeds.

Tabbouleh

Serves 2
Prep 10 minutes
Stand 10 minutes
227 cal per serve

½ cup bulgur (cracked wheat)
2 ripe tomatoes, diced
1 Lebanese cucumber, diced
½ cup freshly chopped parsley
½ cup freshly chopped mint
1 shallot, finely chopped
1 tablespoon extra virgin olive oil
1 tablespoon lemon juice
freshly ground black pepper
⅔ cup plain low-cal yoghurt,
   to serve

This has to be the most refreshing salad ever invented. The trick is to make sure you have the freshest ingredients so you get that wonderful crisp and crunchy texture.

Cover the bulgur with boiling water and leave for 10 minutes. Drain, rinse with cold water and drain again. Place bulgur in a clean tea towel and wring it out to dry.

Place bulgur in a bowl with the remaining ingredients. Season with pepper and toss to combine.

Serve with yoghurt.

Greek salad

My Greek friends would never forgive me if I didn't include a Greek salad in this book, so here it is! Olives can be quite high in calories so if I'm only going to eat a few, I want to be able to taste them. I go for high-quality, deli-style Australian olives.

Place the lettuce on a large platter. Arrange the tomato, capsicum, cucumber, feta, onion and olives on top. Sprinkle with oregano.

Drizzle over the combined vinegar and oil and season with pepper.

Serves 2
Prep 15 minutes
246 cal per serve

1 baby cos lettuce, leaves separated, shredded
3 ripe tomatoes, cut into wedges
½ red capsicum, thinly sliced
1 Lebanese cucumber, sliced
50 g low-cal feta, crumbled
½ small red onion, thinly sliced
⅓ cup kalamata olives
1 teaspoon dried oregano
1 tablespoon cider vinegar
1 tablespoon extra virgin olive oil
freshly ground black pepper

Rocket, grape, walnut and parmesan salad

An amazing summer salad – crunchy, sweet and flavoursome, though it comes with a 'Nut Alert'. Walnuts are very good for you, but are calorie heavyweights (around 25 calories each) so don't be tempted to tuck into a few while you're preparing this!

Combine the rocket, grapes, walnuts and parmesan in a salad bowl. Drizzle over combined olive oil and lemon juice. Season with a little pepper and toss to coat.

Serves 2
Prep 5 minutes
258 cal per serve

4 large handfuls baby rocket
100 g red seedless grapes, halved or quartered
¼ cup walnuts
2 tablespoons shaved parmesan
1 tablespoon extra virgin olive oil
2 teaspoons lemon juice
freshly ground black pepper

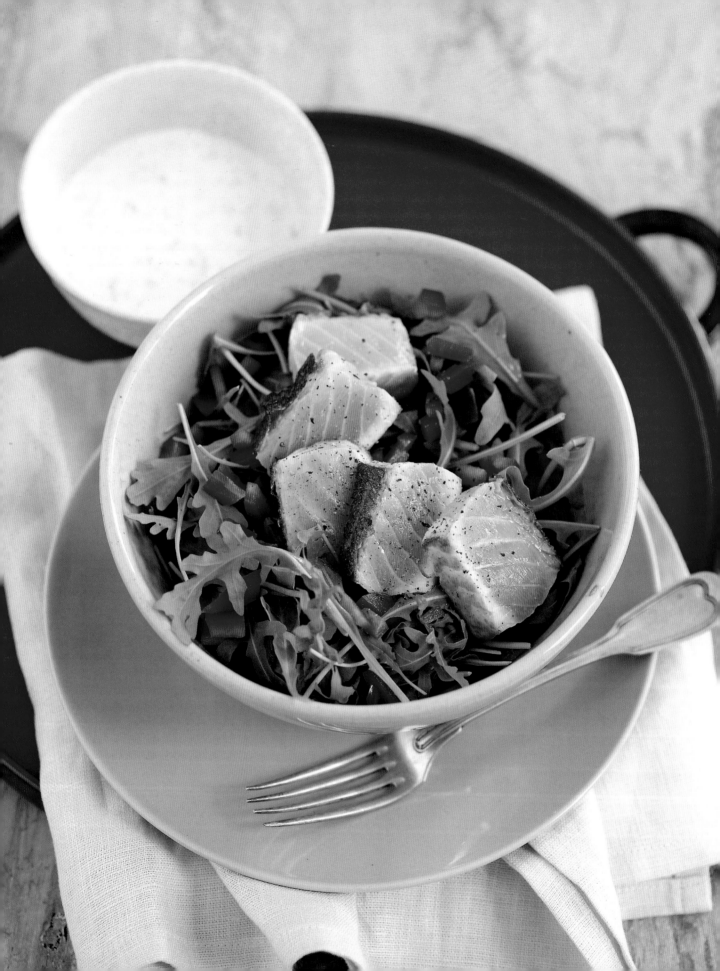

Salmon with tartare sauce and rocket salad

This is another of my staple dishes. Whenever someone starts droning on to me that they don't have time to cook, I use this recipe as an example of a super-quick, super-nutritious and super-delicious meal. Take out the tartare sauce and it takes literally 5 minutes to cook. This is definitely a 'must-learn'!

To make the sauce, combine all the ingredients in a small bowl. Season with pepper.

Lightly spray a non-stick frying pan with oil and heat on medium–high. Cook the salmon skin-side down for 2–3 minutes until crisp. Turn and cook for another 3 minutes until cooked through, but still slightly pink inside.

Meanwhile, combine the rocket and capsicum. Serve the salmon with the rocket salad and tartare sauce.

Tips

- Choose your fish carefully – don't get fillets that are too thick as they won't cook in the middle without burning the yummy skin.
- The tartare sauce recipe is 84 calories all up.

Variation

- This is delicious with other fish, too, but avoid less environmentally responsible species like Atlantic salmon and ocean trout.

Serves 2
Prep 15 minutes
Cook 5 minutes
288 cal per serve

2 × 150 g salmon fillets
4 handfuls rocket
1 red capsicum, thinly sliced

tartare sauce
½ cup plain low-cal yoghurt
½ shallot, finely chopped
2 teaspoons freshly chopped dill
2 teaspoons lemon juice
1 teaspoon chopped capers
freshly ground black pepper

Salmon with char-grilled asparagus and tomato salad

Serves 2
Prep 10 minutes
Cook 10 minutes
269 cal per serve

---

olive oil spray
1 bunch asparagus
300 g cherry tomatoes
1 small oak-leaf lettuce, leaves
    separated and washed
2 tablespoons freshly shredded
    basil
2 teaspoons balsamic vinegar
2 × 150 g salmon steaks

Asparagus is one of those underestimated vegetables from the same family as leeks, onions and garlic. It's loaded with folate and vitamins, and best of all, 100 grams of asparagus is only 24 calories. Store it in the fridge in a glass with an inch of water in the bottom. Your top choice for salmon? Australian salmon, of course!

Lightly spray a char-grill pan with oil and heat on medium–high. Grill the asparagus for 4 minutes. Add the tomatoes and grill for another 4 minutes until they are just tender and lightly charred. Cut the asparagus into chunks and combine with the tomatoes, lettuce, basil and vinegar in a bowl. Toss to coat.

Meanwhile, char-grill the salmon for 5–6 minutes, depending on thickness, until lightly charred and still pink inside. Serve the salmon with the salad.

Tip
● Heat wilts salad leaves, so let the asparagus and tomatoes cool for a few minutes and toss them through the salad just before serving.

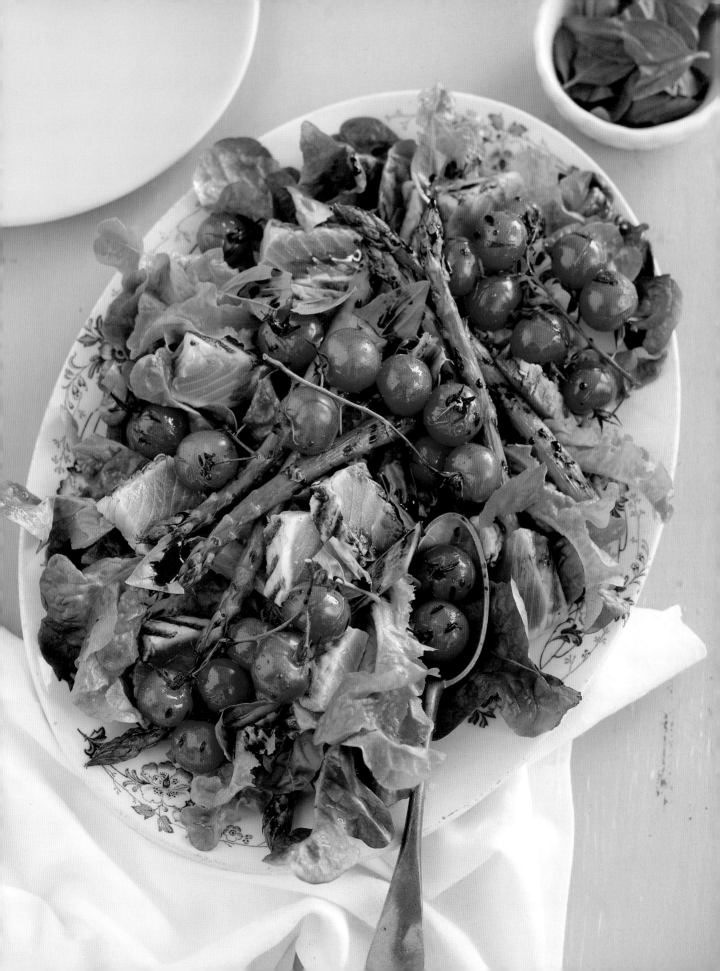

Niçoise salad

Serves 2
Prep 15 minutes
Cook 15 minutes
265 cal per serve

100 g new potatoes
50 g green beans, blanched
1 small oak-leaf lettuce, leaves
    separated and washed
1 hard-boiled egg, quartered
185 g can tuna in springwater,
    drained and flaked
1 red capsicum, thinly sliced
2 tomatoes, cut into wedges
3 anchovy fillets, halved
    lengthways
4 kalamata olives, pitted and
    halved
1 tablespoon red wine vinegar
2 teaspoons extra virgin olive oil
2 teaspoons Dijon mustard
1 garlic clove, crushed
freshly ground black pepper

Don't be put off by the long list of ingredients – this salad is brilliant!
It's low in calories yet really filling, and it's unbelievably tasty thanks to
the anchovies, red wine vinegar and kalamata olives.

Place the potatoes in a saucepan of lightly salted water on medium–
high heat. Bring to the boil and cook for 10–15 minutes until tender.
Add the green beans 2 minutes before the end of the cooking time.
Drain. Cool the beans in cold water, then drain again. Halve the
potatoes when they are cool enough to handle.

Arrange the lettuce, egg, tuna, capsicum, tomatoes, potatoes
and beans in a bowl. Top with the anchovy and olives.

Whisk together the vinegar, olive oil, mustard and garlic in a
small bowl. Season to taste with pepper and drizzle over the salad.

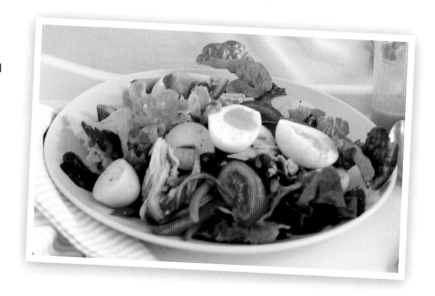

Risoni, tuna, baby spinach and snowpea salad with lemon and dill

Canned tuna is a product I buy carefully, because I want to be sure that it has been caught as responsibly as possible, plus I don't want it to look like cat food when I open the tin. Go for a nice flaky tuna that comes in chunks to get the most out of this great salad. Pasta salads tend to be a bit more filling than leaf salads, so this is a good lunchtime choice.

Cook the risoni in a saucepan of boiling, lightly salted water according to the packet directions. Add the peas and snowpeas 1 minute before the end of the cooking time. Drain and rinse under cold water. Drain again.

Combine the risoni, peas, snowpeas, lemon zest and juice, garlic, oil, capers and dill in a bowl. Toss through the tuna and baby spinach leaves to serve.

Serves 2
Prep 10 minutes
Cook 10 minutes
304 cal per serve

½ cup risoni
½ cup frozen peas
50 g snowpeas, trimmed and thinly sliced on the diagonal
1 lemon, grated zest and juice
1 garlic clove, crushed
2 teaspoons extra virgin olive oil
2 teaspoons baby capers, rinsed
2 teaspoons chopped dill
185 g can tuna in springwater, drained and flaked
2 large handfuls baby spinach leaves

Chicken with fennel, cabbage, radish and cranberry coleslaw

Serves 2
Prep 15 minutes
Cook 10 minutes
290 cal per serve

---

olive oil spray
220 g chicken breast fillet, trimmed
freshly ground black pepper

coleslaw
1 large bulb fennel, thinly sliced
150 g cabbage, thinly sliced
6 radishes, cut into matchsticks
⅓ cup low-cal plain yoghurt
1 tablespoon lemon juice
1½ teaspoons horseradish
¼ cup dried cranberries, chopped

Fennel has to be one of the most underused vegies in this country, yet it has a most exotic flavour. I use it in a lot of my salads. This is yet another dish where I will cook a bit extra for sandwiches or salads later in the week.

Lightly spray a non-stick frying pan with oil and heat on medium. Season the chicken with pepper and cook for 5–6 minutes each side until browned and cooked through. Cover and set aside.

To make the coleslaw, combine the fennel, cabbage and radish in a bowl. In a separate bowl, combine the yoghurt, lemon juice and horseradish, then toss half of this with the vegetables.

Cut the chicken into thin slices. Drizzle the remaining dressing over the coleslaw and sprinkle with the cranberries. Serve the coleslaw with the sliced chicken.

Tip
• To make extra coleslaw for sandwiches, simply double the ingredients and store leftovers in an airtight container in the fridge.

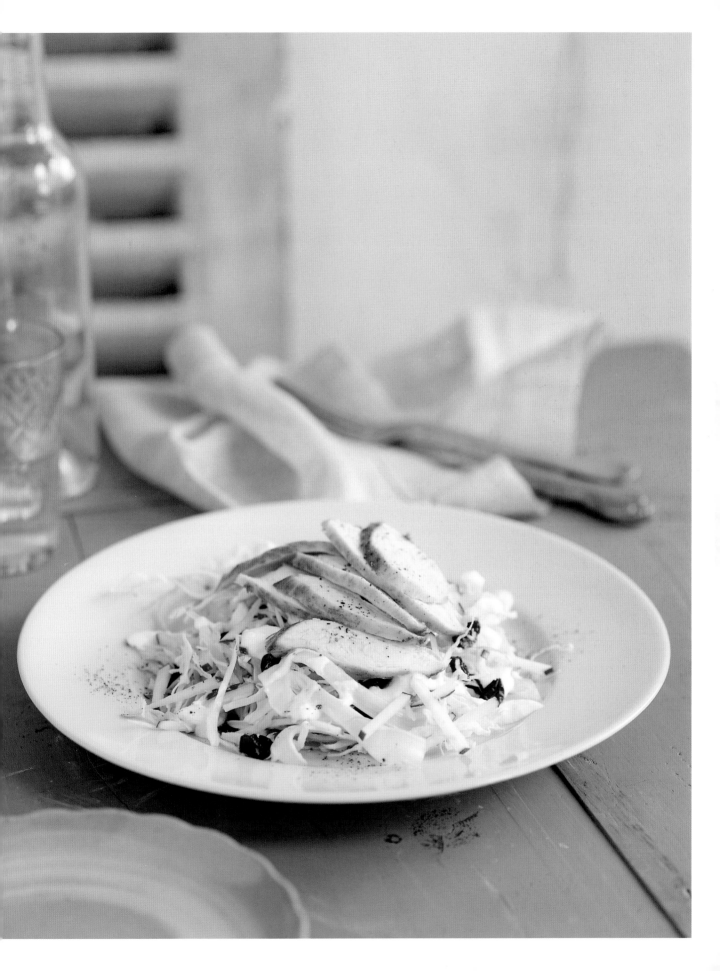

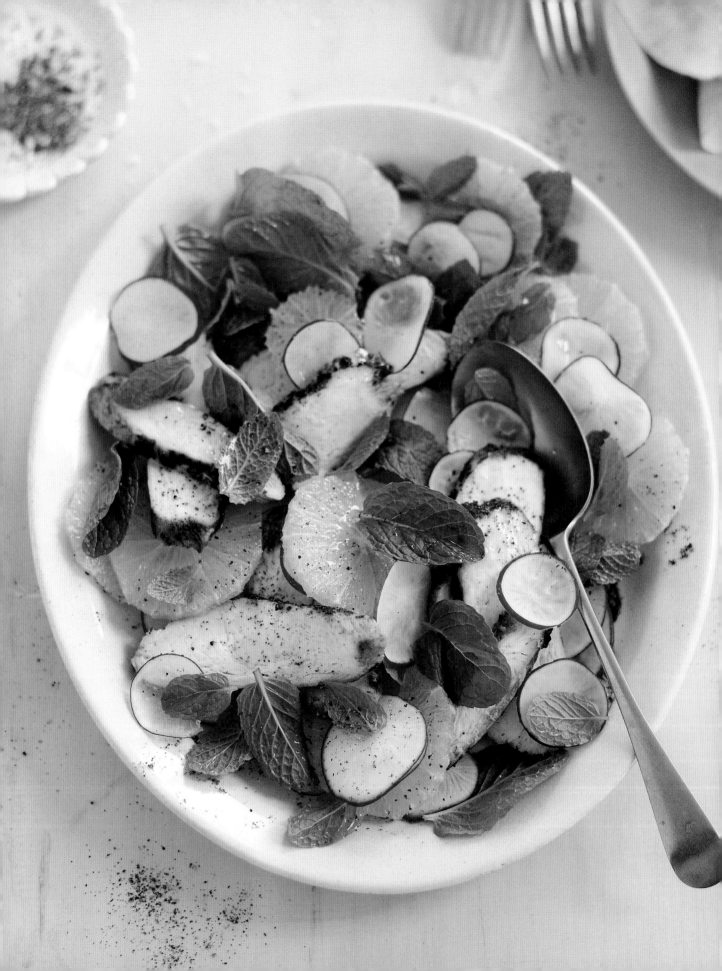

Moroccan chicken, orange and mint salad

I adore the orange and mint in this dish. Don't be freaked out by the Moroccan spices – you can buy them ready made, or if you want to, prepare them yourself (see note at end of recipe).

Coat the chicken with the Moroccan seasoning. Lightly spray a non-stick frying pan with oil and heat on medium. Cook the chicken for 5–6 minutes each side until browned and cooked through. Cover and rest for 2 minutes before thinly slicing.

Meanwhile, peel the oranges and remove the pith. Halve and slice thinly, reserving any juice. Combine the orange slices and juice in a shallow dish with the radishes, mixed leaves, mint and olive oil. Add the chicken and any juices, and toss gently.

Tip
- To make your own **Moroccan seasoning**, mix 2 teaspoons each of ground nutmeg, cumin and coriander, 1 teaspoon each of ground ginger and turmeric, and ½ teaspoon each of paprika and cinnamon. Store in an airtight container.

Variation
- Segment the oranges for a different look, or use mandarins (they are lower in calories).

Serves 2
Prep 15 minutes
Cook 15 minutes
266 cal per serve

220 g chicken breast fillet, trimmed
3 teaspoons Moroccan seasoning (see below)
olive oil spray
2 small oranges
4 radishes, thinly sliced
3 handfuls mixed salad leaves
½ cup mint leaves
2 teaspoons extra virgin olive oil

Chicken salad with baby spinach, blackberries, apple, feta and walnut

Serves 2
Prep 15 minutes
Cook 10 minutes
348 cal per serve

olive oil spray
200 g chicken breast fillet, trimmed
freshly ground black pepper
4 handfuls baby spinach
1 small green apple, cored and cut into matchsticks
1 small celery stick, sliced
1 tablespoon white balsamic vinegar
2 teaspoons extra virgin olive oil
50 g blackberries
2 tablespoons chopped walnuts
30 g low-cal feta, crumbled

It's the variety of ingredients that make this dish a cracker! As with all grilled chicken dishes, think about making extra for other salads and sandwiches. The blackberries give a nice sweet touch, but you can try raspberries or blueberries too.

Preheat the grill to high. Line a baking sheet with foil and lightly spray with oil. Place the chicken on the prepared sheet and season to taste with pepper. Cook the chicken 10 cm away from the grill for 5 minutes, then turn and cook the other side until the chicken is browned and cooked through. Cover and rest for 2 minutes before thinly slicing.

Meanwhile, combine the spinach, apple and celery in a bowl. Add the vinegar and oil and toss to coat. Divide the salad between 2 serving plates and top with the sliced chicken. Scatter over the blackberries, walnuts and feta to serve.

Tip
• Walnuts are 25 calories *each*, so no nibbling or you'll blow your calorie count out the window.

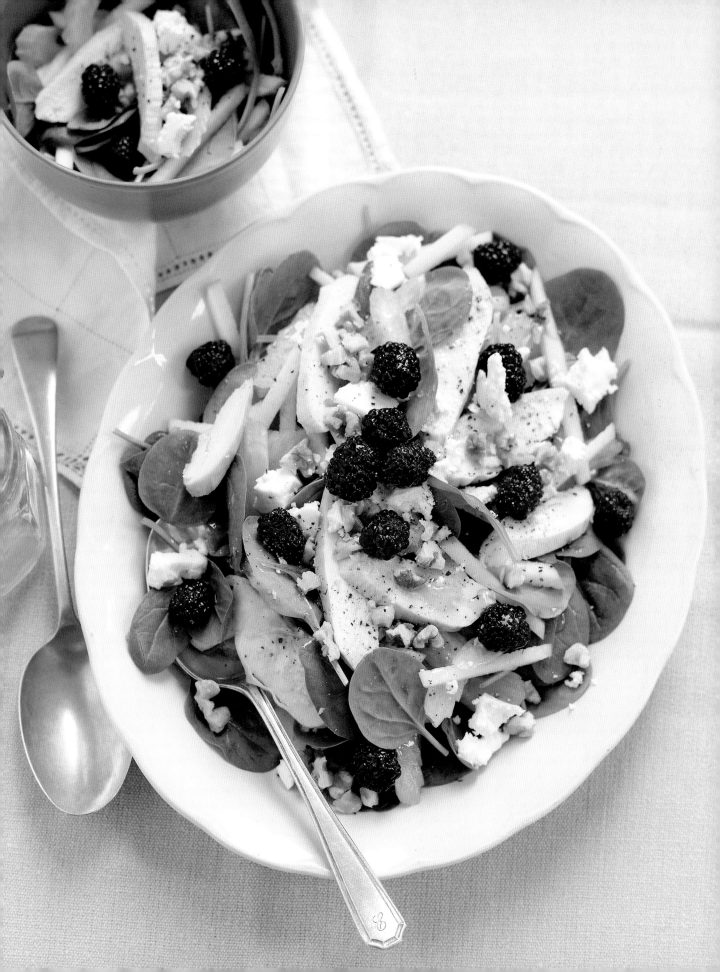

Coleslaw

Serves 2
Prep 15 minutes
185 cal per serve

200 g green cabbage, finely
    shredded
1 large red capsicum, cut into
    thin strips
1 large carrot, coarsely grated
2 shallots, finely sliced
¾ cup plain low-cal yoghurt
2 teaspoons Dijon mustard
freshly ground black pepper

Everyone's favourite at a barbecue, but mine is made with low-calorie plain yoghurt instead of the sugary slop marketed as coleslaw dressing. If you like a bit of bite in your coleslaw, a dash or two of tabasco will kick it on a bit. Use any left over coleslaw for a lunchtime wrap.

Combine the cabbage, capsicum, carrot and shallots in a large salad bowl. Combine the yoghurt, mustard and 1½ tablespoons water in a small bowl and season with pepper to taste.

Add the dressing to the salad and toss well to mix. Cover and chill before serving.

Tip
• To make extra for sandwiches, simply double your ingredients and store leftovers in an airtight container in the fridge.

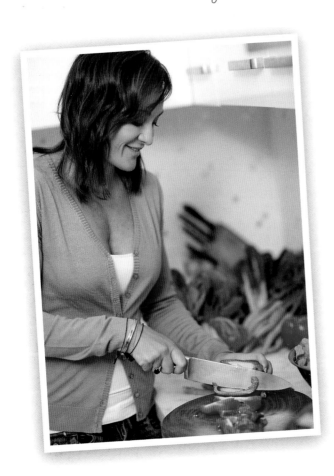

Poached chicken, mixed bean and ginger salad

I love how colourful this salad looks when it's served. Poaching the chicken is not only easy, but keeps the chicken super moist and yummy. Sometimes I serve this salad without the chicken as a side dish in summer – it's excellent for barbecues and entertaining.

Place the chicken in a small saucepan and cover with water. Bring to the boil. Reduce the heat and simmer for 5 minutes. Remove from the heat and leave the chicken in the cooking liquid for 10 minutes to cook through. Remove the chicken from the liquid. When cool enough to handle, shred the chicken. Cool the chicken stock and refrigerate or freeze for another use.

Meanwhile, cook the beans in a large saucepan of boiling, lightly salted water for 3 minutes until just tender. Drain and rinse immediately in cold water. Drain again.

Combine the vinegar, oil and ginger in a small bowl. Place the beans, tomatoes, spinach, shallots and chicken in a salad bowl. Drizzle over the dressing and toss to coat.

Tip
- Poach an extra breast fillet for making sandwiches through the week.

Serves 2
Prep 10 minutes
Cook 15 minutes
324 cal per serve

220 g chicken breast fillet, trimmed
150 g yellow beans, trimmed
150 g green beans, trimmed
1 tablespoon white balsamic vinegar
2 teaspoons olive oil
1 teaspoon grated ginger
150 g cherry tomatoes, halved
4 handfuls baby spinach
2 shallot bulbs, thinly sliced

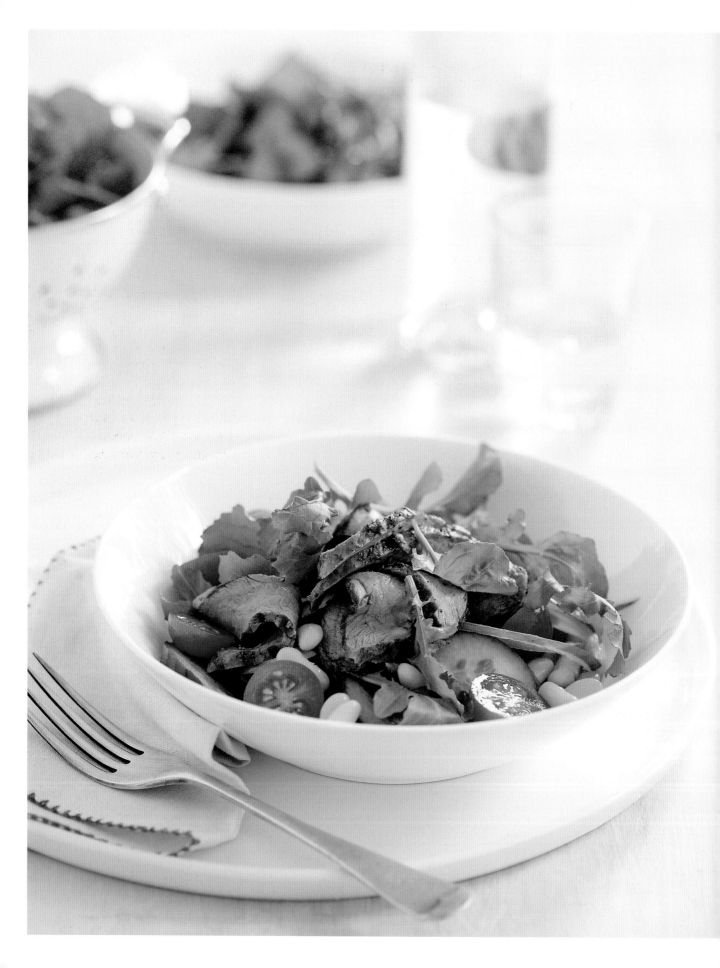

Lamb, cannellini bean and rocket salad

This one is really lovely on a warm summer's day. I like the contrast of flavours and textures – the beans have that nice earthy flavour, the lamb is sweet and rich, and the peppery rocket gives a bitey finish.

Lightly spray a char-grill pan with olive oil and heat on medium–high. Season the lamb with pepper. Cook for 2 minutes each side until browned and still lightly pink inside. Remove the pan from the heat and add the lemon juice and garlic. Turn the meat to coat. Cover and rest for 5 minutes.

Meanwhile, combine the beans, rocket, cucumber, tomatoes, red onion and olive oil in a bowl. Slice the lamb thickly and drizzle the meat juices over the salad. Toss the salad and serve topped with the lamb slices.

Tip

- To use dried cannellini beans, cook ⅔ cup dried beans according to the packet directions and use as described above. (There are usually a couple of options for cooking dried beans: an 'overnight soak' method, and a 'rapid boil' method.)

Serves 2
Prep 15 minutes
Cook 5 minutes
312 cal per serve

olive oil spray
220 g lamb backstrap
freshly ground black pepper
½ lemon, juice
1 garlic clove, crushed
400 g can cannellini beans, drained and rinsed
4 handfuls rocket
1 Lebanese cucumber, sliced
200 g cherry tomatoes, halved
¼ red onion, thinly sliced
2 teaspoons extra virgin olive oil

Thai beef salad

Serves 2
Prep 10 minutes
Cook 5 minutes
225 cal per serve

250 g cherry tomatoes, quartered
1 Lebanese cucumber, cut into
  chunks
30 g Asian salad mix
¼ red onion, thinly sliced
½ cup mint leaves
½ cup coriander leaves
1 long red chilli, thinly sliced
2 tablespoons lime juice
1 tablespoon fish sauce
1 teaspoon palm sugar
vegetable oil spray
220 g beef rump steak, trimmed
freshly ground black pepper

Low calories, gorgeous flavours and 15 minutes to prepare *and* cook make this a gold-star meal! You can make it as hot as you like depending on your choice of chilli – the little bird's-eye chillies have the mightiest kick. And don't worry if the beef seems a bit rare, the lime juice will finish off the cooking process. Packaged 'Asian salad' mixes can be found at the supermarket and contain green leaves such as tatsoi, mizuna, baby rocket, Chinese cabbage and pea shoots.

Combine the tomatoes, cucumber, Asian salad, red onion, mint, coriander and chilli in a large bowl. Mix the lime juice, fish sauce and palm sugar in a small bowl until the sugar has dissolved.

Lightly spray a char-grill pan with vegetable oil and heat on high. Season the steak with pepper. Cook for 1 minute each side until well browned. Cover loosely and rest in a warm place (e.g. on the stovetop or in a low oven) for 5 minutes before thinly slicing.

Add the beef to the salad, then pour over the dressing and toss to coat.

Variation

• This salad rocks when you substitute kangaroo fillet for the beef. Cook and prepare it the same way as the beef.

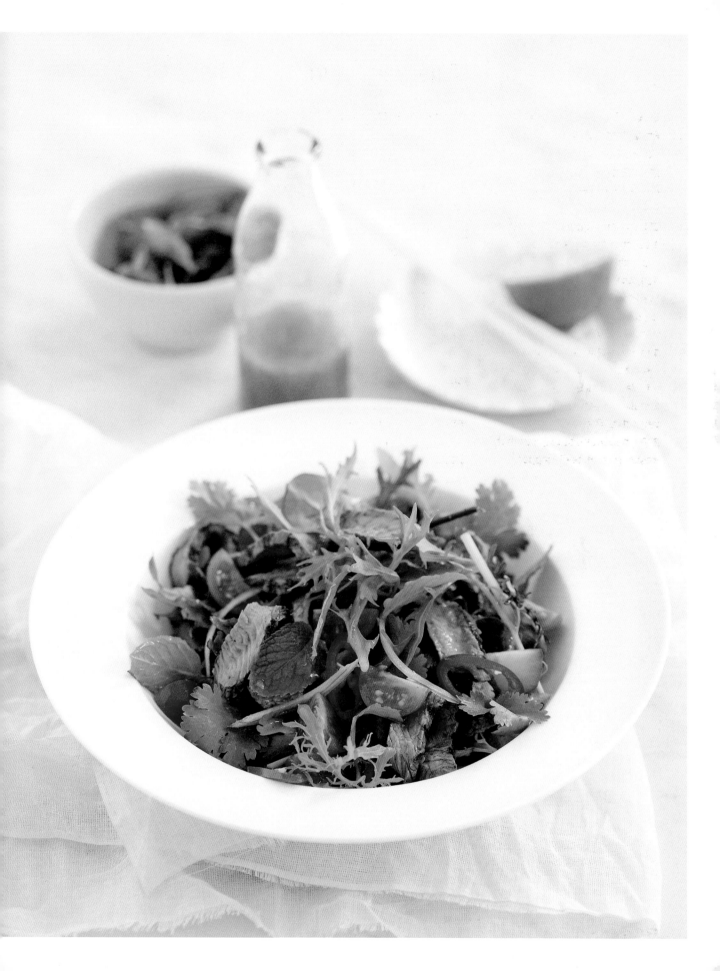

Kangaroo and mint salad with char-grilled zucchini and capsicum

Serves 2
Prep 10 minutes
Marinate 15 minutes
Cook 15 minutes
276 cal per serve

220 g kangaroo fillet, cut into strips
2 garlic cloves, sliced
¼ cup mint leaves, torn
1 tablespoon extra virgin olive oil
freshly ground black pepper
olive oil spray
1 large red capsicum, halved and seeded
3 zucchini, cut into ribbons (see tip)
2 tablespoons white balsamic vinegar

If you are a newcomer to the taste of this amazing meat, marinating is the way to go. And as for char-grilling vegies, I cannot begin to tell you how much I love this method of cooking. This is where an olive oil spray is priceless – you can coat the vegies without drowning them. I always make extra for sandwiches the next day.

Combine the kangaroo, the garlic, 1 tablespoon of the mint and 1 teaspoon of the oil in a bowl. Season with pepper and toss to coat. Marinate for 15 minutes.

Meanwhile, lightly spray a char-grill pan with olive oil and heat on high. Cook the capsicum, skin-side down, for 5 minutes until the skin is black. Place in a plastic bag to sweat for 10 minutes. Remove and discard the skin. Cut the capsicum into strips.

Meanwhile, char-grill the zucchini in batches for 1–2 minutes until lightly charred and tender but not sloppy. Combine the zucchini, capsicum, vinegar and remaining oil and mint in a shallow dish. Toss to coat.

Lightly spray a non-stick frying pan with oil and heat on high. Cook the kangaroo in 2 batches for 1–2 minutes until browned. Toss through the salad.

Tip
- To cut the zucchini into ribbons, first quarter them lengthways. Then, using a Y-shaped vegetable peeler, cut each quarter into thin, long strips. If you prefer, simply halve or quarter the zucchini and slice very thinly using a sharp knife.

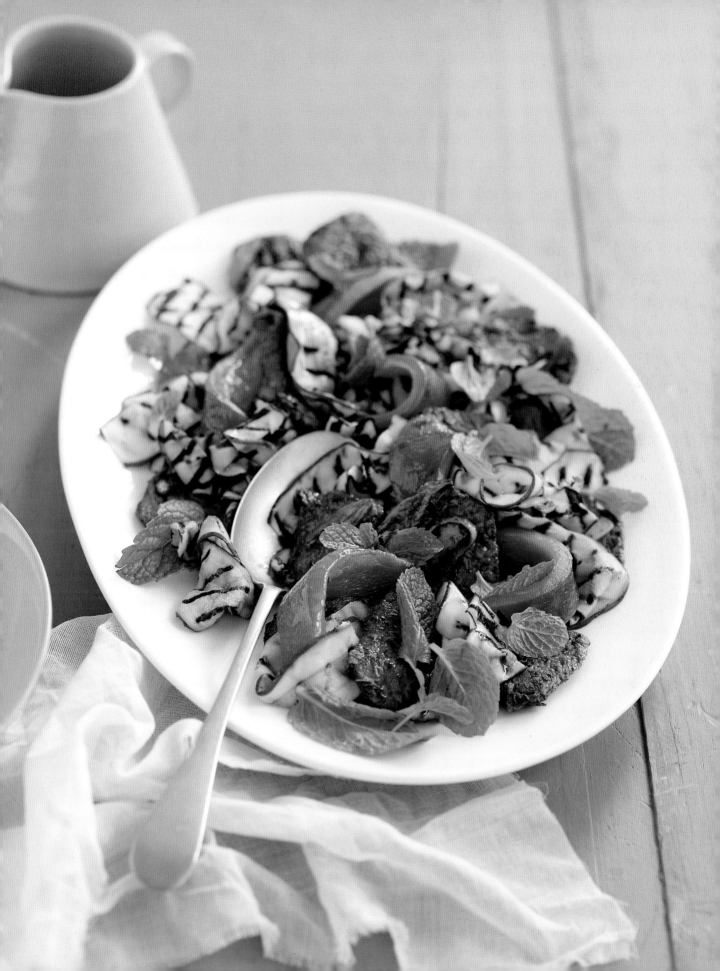

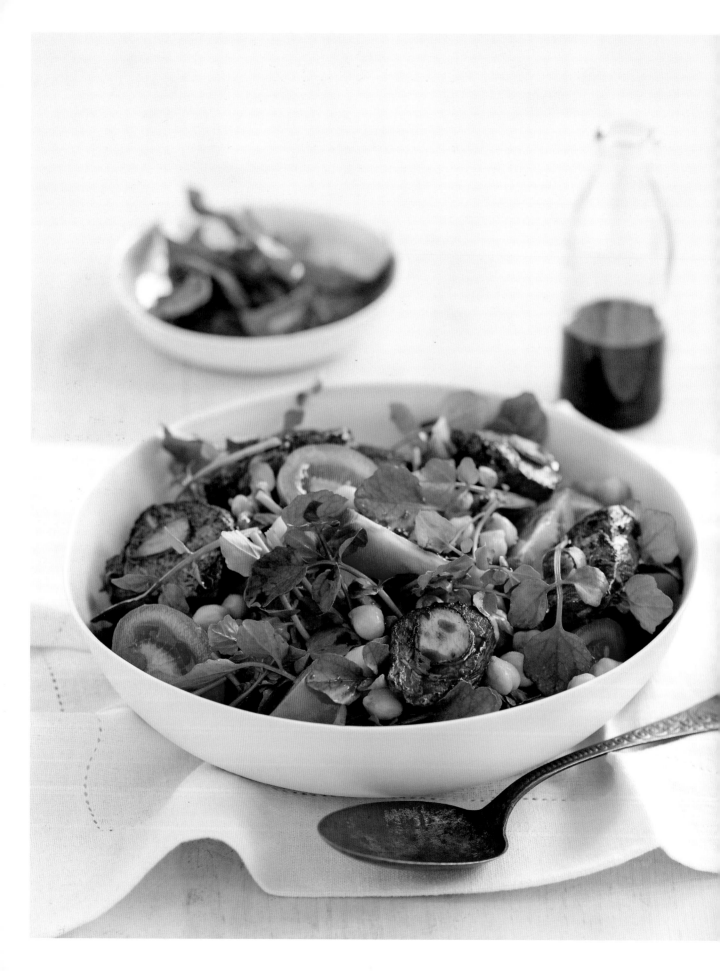

Kangaroo with watercress, chickpea, tomato and basil salad

Kangaroo has so much to offer – it's low in fat, completely organic and very affordable. To make the most of this underrated meat, it needs to be cooked with care. I keep it on the rare side so that it doesn't dry out, and always let it stand before cutting.

Combine the kangaroo, garlic, 2 tablespoons of the basil and 1 teaspoon of the oil in a bowl. Season with pepper and toss to coat. Marinate for 15 minutes.

Meanwhile, combine the watercress, tomato, chickpeas and remaining basil in a salad bowl.

Lightly spray a non-stick frying pan with olive oil and heat on high. Cook the kangaroo for 2 minutes each side until browned and rare. Allow the meat to rest, covered, for 5 minutes before slicing.

Add the vinegar and remaining oil to the salad, season to taste with pepper and toss. Serve the kangaroo with the salad.

Variations

- Try a marinade of 1 tablespoon salt-reduced soy sauce, 1 teaspoon olive oil, 1 chopped shallot, 1 tablespoon lime juice and 1 clove garlic, crushed.
- Another tasty marinade is 1 tablespoon freshly chopped ginger, 1 clove garlic, crushed, 1 tablespoon salt-reduced soy sauce and 1 teaspoon vegetable oil.
- Or try 2 tablespoons Italian tomato sauce, 2 teaspoons Worcestershire sauce and a little lemon juice.

Serves 2
Prep 10 minutes
Marinate 15 minutes
Cook 5 minutes
341 cal per serve

220 g kangaroo fillet, cut into 7 cm pieces
2 garlic cloves, sliced
⅓ cup basil leaves, torn
1 tablespoon extra virgin olive oil
freshly ground black pepper
1 small bunch watercress, leaves picked
3 tomatoes, cut into wedges
300 g can chickpeas, drained and rinsed
olive oil spray
1 tablespoon balsamic vinegar

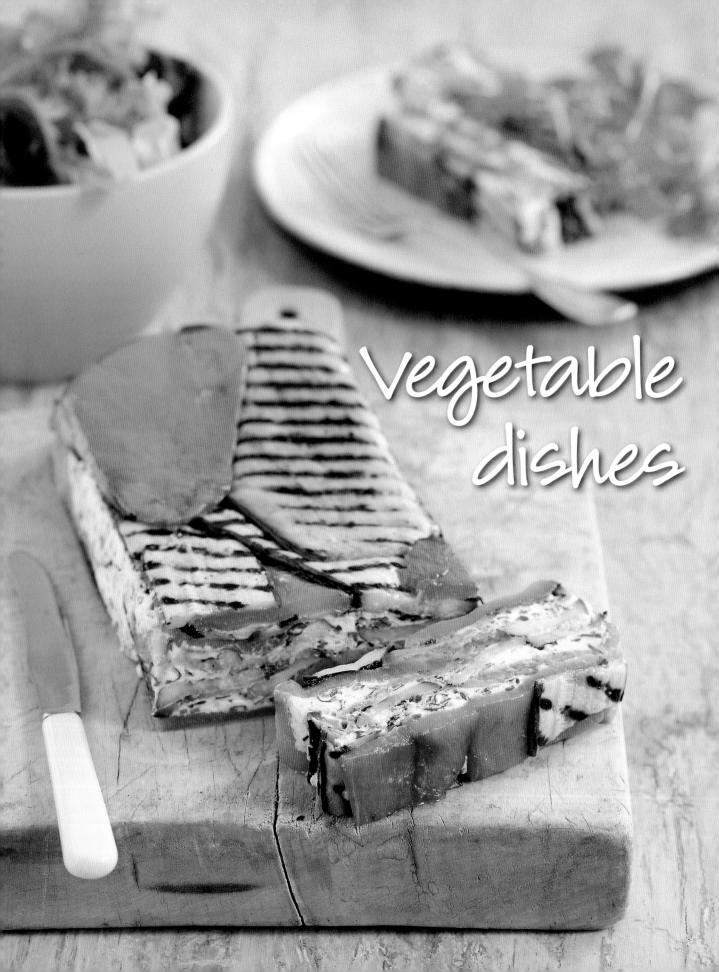

Vegetable
dishes

Char-grilled vegetable terrine

I cook this when I'm having a *MasterChef* moment. Although it looks difficult, it's actually quite easy. There'll be gasps of appreciation when you serve it up!

Preheat the grill to hot. Place the capsicums in a roasting dish and grill for 15 minutes, turning regularly, until the skin is charred. Transfer to a plastic bag and set aside for 15 minutes. Taking care not to burn yourself, remove the capsicums from the bag. Remove and discard the skin, stem, seeds and membrane. Cut into wide strips.

Meanwhile, lightly spray a char-grill pan with olive oil and heat on medium–high. Char-grill the eggplant and zucchini for 1–2 minutes until soft and lightly charred.

Combine the ricotta, basil, chives and olive oil in a bowl. Season with pepper.

Line a 25 cm × 11 cm loaf pan with plastic wrap, leaving enough hanging over the sides to fold over and enclose the terrine. Starting and finishing with vegetables, layer the vegetables and ricotta mixture alternately, seasoning every 2–3 layers and pressing down to flatten. Fold over the plastic wrap to enclose, and refrigerate overnight.

Bring the terrine to room temperature before serving. Slice with a serrated knife and serve with the salad leaves.

Tips
- Don't worry too much about layering the ricotta mixture. Just dollop in a few spoonfuls – when you press down the next layer of vegetables it will spread out.
- Make sure the plastic wrap is tight against the outside of the loaf pan with a minimum of air pockets and wrinkles – that way it will look fabulous when served.
- Make some extra char-grilled vegies for sandwiches.

Serves 4
Prep 25 minutes
Cook 15 minutes
Chill overnight
221 cal per serve

2 large red capsicums
olive oil spray
1 large eggplant, thinly sliced lengthways
4 zucchini, thinly sliced lengthways
1 cup low-cal ricotta
⅓ cup freshly chopped basil
1 bunch chives, finely chopped
1 tablespoon extra virgin olive oil
freshly ground black pepper
4 handfuls mixed salad leaves, to serve

Roasted vegetables and tofu with rosemary

Serves 2
Prep 10 minutes
Cook 1 hour
343 cal per serve

250 g butternut pumpkin,
    unpeeled and cut into chunks
1 medium eggplant, cut into
    chunks
1 parsnip, peeled and cut into
    chunks
2 teaspoons olive oil
freshly ground black pepper
1 sprig rosemary, leaves only
1 small sweet potato, peeled
    and cut into chunks
150 g firm tofu, drained and
    cut into cubes
4 garlic cloves, unpeeled

This is another staple recipe that you need to be skilled in – the variations are endless, and the oven time means you get to do some chores while it's cooking. Definitely a 'must-learn'! Don't be put off if some of these vegies aren't your favourites – when vegetables are roasted they take on a unique flavour and you might find you like them!

Preheat the oven to 210°C. Arrange the pumpkin, eggplant and parsnip in a single layer in a large (35 cm × 25 cm) ovenproof dish. Drizzle with the oil, season with pepper, and sprinkle with the rosemary. Toss to coat. Roast for 20 minutes.

Add the sweet potato, tofu and garlic and roast for another 20 minutes. Toss the vegetables, then cook for another 20 minutes or until soft.

Tip

• It's important that the vegetables and tofu are in a single layer in the baking dish, or they will steam rather than roast.

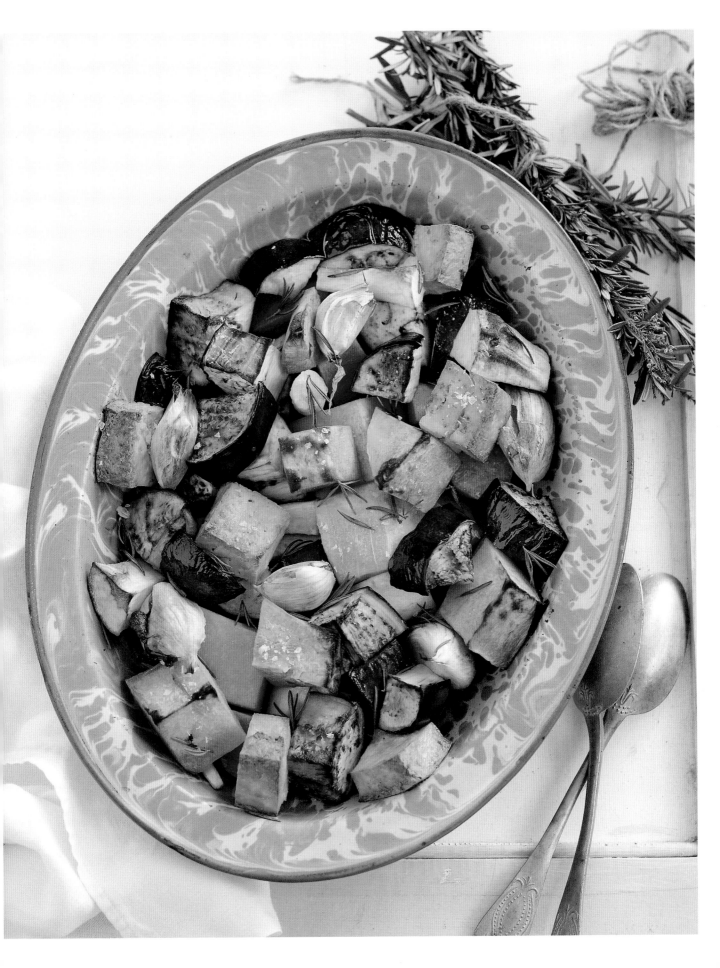

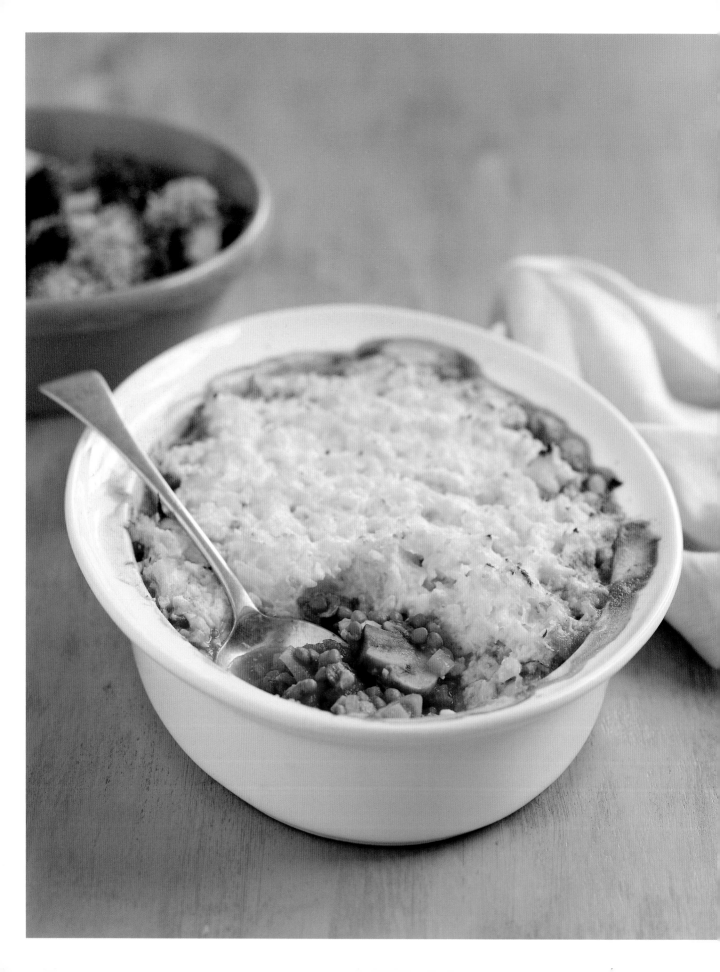

Lentil shepherd's pie with steamed broccoli

Just like a traditional shepherd's pie, but without the fatty mince and mashed spuds our mums used to make it with. This is a weekend dish, but using canned lentils might cut down the prep time so you can enjoy it during the week. I've doubled the quantities so you can reheat for another meal or serve a family.

Place the lentils, whole onion and bay leaf in a saucepan. Cover with 2 cups of water and bring to the boil. Gently boil for 40 minutes until the lentils are tender. Drain and discard the onion and bay leaf.

Meanwhile, place the cauliflower in a steamer basket over simmering water. Steam for 15 minutes until very soft. Transfer to a bowl and mash with the ricotta to make a coarse puree.

Lightly spray a frying pan with oil. Cook chopped onion, carrot, mushroom and garlic for 8 minutes, stirring until softened and lightly browned. Stir through the tomatoes, drained lentils and ¼ cup water. Season with pepper then spoon the mixture into a 32 cm × 20 cm ovenproof dish. Top with the cauliflower mash and sprinkle the parmesan over the top. Bake for 30 minutes until the cheese is golden.

Serve with steamed broccoli.

Tip
- To make this on a weeknight, use a 400 g can of lentils to speed things up. Drain and rinse before adding to onion mixture.

Variation
- Try it with a sweet potato topping instead. Peel 500 g sweet potato and cut into chunks. Steam until tender (about 10 minutes) and mash (348 calories per serve).

Serves 4
Prep 20 minutes
Cook 1 hour 10 minutes
290 cal per serve

½ cup dried brown lentils
2 onions, 1 whole, 1 chopped
1 bay leaf
500 g cauliflower, broken into florets
⅓ cup low-cal ricotta
olive oil spray
1 large carrot, diced
150 g mixed mushrooms, halved depending on size
1 garlic clove, crushed
400 g can diced tomatoes
freshly ground black pepper
⅓ cup grated parmesan
400 g steamed broccoli, to serve

Ratatouille

Serves 4
Prep 10 minutes
Cook 1 hour 25 minutes
247 cal per serve

4 garlic cloves, peeled
1 tablespoon olive oil
1 onion, chopped
3 medium eggplants, cut
   into chunks
3 large zucchini, cut into chunks
3 red capsicums, cut into chunks
400 g can diced tomatoes
5 sprigs thyme
1 bay leaf
½ teaspoon dried oregano
4 slices wholegrain bread,
   to serve

Ratatouille is one of my favourite movies, as well as one of my favourite meals! Although it takes a bit of time to cook, it's well worth it. Make plenty, as it freezes well and can save you lots of time in the long run. It can also be used as a base for other meals, which earns it a double thumbs-up from me.

Crush 3 of the garlic cloves and set the other one aside.

Heat the oil in a large, heavy-based saucepan over medium heat, then cook the onion and crushed garlic for 5 minutes, stirring, until softened. Add the eggplant and cook for 5 minutes. Add the zucchini, capsicum, tomato, herbs and ½ cup water. Bring to a simmer. Cook, covered, on a low heat for 1¼ hours until the vegetables are tender.

Just before serving, toast the bread and rub it with the reserved garlic clove. Serve the ratatouille with the garlic toast.

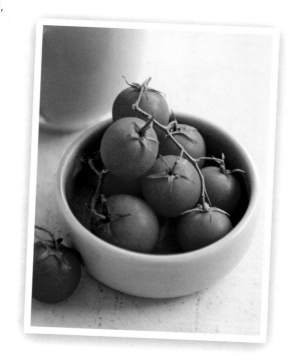

Vegetable stacks with tofu

The great thing about cooking vegetable dishes is the number of variations you can try with different vegies, herbs and spices. This dish takes a bit of preparation, so it's probably a weekender, but it's a fantastic winter meal and looks really dramatic when you serve it up. Any leftovers will make yummy sandwiches for weekday lunches.

Serves 2 (4 stacks)
Prep 15 minutes
Cook 25 minutes
341 cal per serve

olive oil spray
1 small onion, cut into 4 slices
½ medium eggplant, cut into
  4 × 2 cm rounds
½ medium sweet potato, cut
  into 4 × 2 cm rounds
4 large field mushrooms
4 garlic cloves, peeled
2 teaspoons finely chopped
  thyme leaves
1½ teaspoons caraway seeds
freshly ground black pepper
1 bunch spinach, trimmed and
  washed
150 g firm tofu, cut into 4 slices
4 handfuls salad leaves, to serve

Preheat the oven to 220°C. Line a large baking sheet with baking paper and lightly spray with olive oil.

Lightly spray a non-stick frying pan and heat on medium. Cook the onion slices for 2 minutes each side until softened. Meanwhile, place the eggplant and sweet potato in a steamer basket and steam for 4 minutes over simmering water until slightly softened.

Place the onion, eggplant, sweet potato, mushrooms and garlic on the baking sheet. Lightly spray with oil. Sprinkle over the thyme and caraway seeds and season to taste with pepper. Roast for 20 minutes.

Meanwhile, steam the spinach and the tofu separately for 1 minute each. Drain the spinach well and coarsely chop.

To assemble, drain the mushrooms before placing 2 on each serving plate. Mash the garlic and spread on the mushrooms. Top with the spinach, eggplant, tofu, sweet potato and onion to make a stack.

Serve with the salad leaves.

Variations

• My favourite way to serve these stacks is with a dollop of spicy tamarind chutney on top – O.M.G! You can find tamarind chutney at your supermarket or Asian grocery store.
• Try replacing the thyme and caraway seeds with ground cumin, rosemary and paprika.

Zesty tofu and shiitake mushroom stir-fry

Serves 2
Prep 15 minutes
Cook 10 minutes
295 cal per serve

1 bunch asparagus, trimmed
   and cut into 3 cm lengths
2 teaspoons vegetable oil
150 g firm tofu, drained and
   cut into cubes
1 onion, thinly sliced
150 g shiitake mushrooms, sliced
10 cm stalk lemongrass, finely
   chopped
1 garlic clove, crushed
1 tablespoon low-GI sugar
200 g sugarsnap peas, trimmed
2 kaffir lime leaves, finely
   shredded
2 tablespoons freshly squeezed
   lime juice
salt and freshly ground
   black pepper

Mushrooms are good – but shiitake mushrooms are great. They have been shown to have many medicinal and healing properties, and are particularly good for your liver, heart and immune system. Plus, they taste fab! I love this recipe because it's spicy and quick to cook – and it's good for my health. It's a perfect light, evening meal.

Blanch the asparagus in a pan of boiling water for 1 minute. Drain.

Heat the oil in a non-stick wok over high heat. Stir-fry the tofu for 3 minutes until golden. Remove from the wok.

Heat the wok again. Stir-fry the onion for 2 minutes until softened. Add the mushrooms, lemongrass and garlic and stir-fry until fragrant. Then add the sugar and 2 tablespoons water and stir-fry until slightly caramelised. Add the peas, asparagus and ¼ cup water. Stir-fry for 3 minutes until tender. Return the tofu to the wok and stir-fry for another minute until hot. Sprinkle with the kaffir lime leaves and drizzle with the lime juice. Season to taste with salt and pepper and serve immediately.

Mixed vegetable and tofu stir-fry

Here is the meal that Billy and I cook more than any other. Get skilled with this one and you'll always be able to prepare a nutritious calorie-controlled meal at the drop of a hat. The trap for new players is not to cook the vegies to death, but to keep them slightly crunchy.

Serves 2
Prep 10 minutes
Cook 10 minutes
291 cal per serve

400 g cauliflower, broken
  into florets
1 tablespoon vegetable oil
150 g firm tofu, drained and
  cut into cubes
150 g green beans, trimmed
1 yellow capsicum, thinly sliced
1 tablespoon freshly grated ginger
1 tablespoon hoisin sauce
2 teaspoons chilli garlic sauce
2 teaspoons oyster sauce

Blanch the cauliflower in a saucepan of boiling, lightly salted water for 1 minute. Drain.

Heat half the oil in a non-stick wok over a high heat. Stir-fry the tofu for 3 minutes until golden. Remove from the wok.

Heat the remaining oil in the wok over medium–high heat. Stir-fry the cauliflower, beans and capsicum for 4 minutes until just tender. Add the ginger, sauces and 2 tablespoons water. Stir-fry until the vegetables are well coated. Return the tofu to the wok and toss gently. Serve immediately.

Variations

• You can use a host of different vegies with this one – broccolini, red and green capsicum, bok choy, asparagus and shallots, to name a few.

• If you don't have the hoisin, chilli or oyster sauces you can still make this dish. Simply use a few slivers of freshly sliced chilli and a splash of soy sauce.

• Try smoked tofu instead of ordinary tofu – it adds an extra flavour hit.

Mixed vegetable stir-fry with oyster sauce

Serves 2
Prep 15 minutes
Cook 10 minutes
239 cal per serve

1 tablespoon vegetable oil
1 bunch broccolini, stems
    quartered lengthways, cut
    into chunks
2 medium carrots, halved
    lengthways and sliced on
    the diagonal
150 g mixed mushrooms (shiitake,
    Swiss brown, enoki), sliced
3 garlic cloves, crushed
3 shallots, thinly sliced on
    the diagonal
400 g wombok (Chinese cabbage),
    coarsely shredded
2 tablespoons oyster sauce
1 tablespoon salt-reduced soy
    sauce

This is similar to the mixed vegetable and tofu stir-fry (page 119) and just as delicious – it simply uses garlic and a greater variety of vegies. As always, go easy on the sauces as this is where your calories and salt content can mount up.

Heat half the oil in a non-stick wok over high heat. Stir-fry the broccolini for 2 minutes. Add the carrot and stir-fry for another 3 minutes until just tender. Remove the vegetables from the wok.

Heat the remaining oil and stir-fry the mushrooms, garlic and half the shallots for 2 minutes until the mushrooms have browned. Return the broccolini and carrot to the wok with the wombok and sauces. Stir-fry for 2 minutes until the cabbage has just wilted.

Garnish with the remaining shallots to serve.

Tip

- If you can't get wombok, try using choy sum or bok choy.

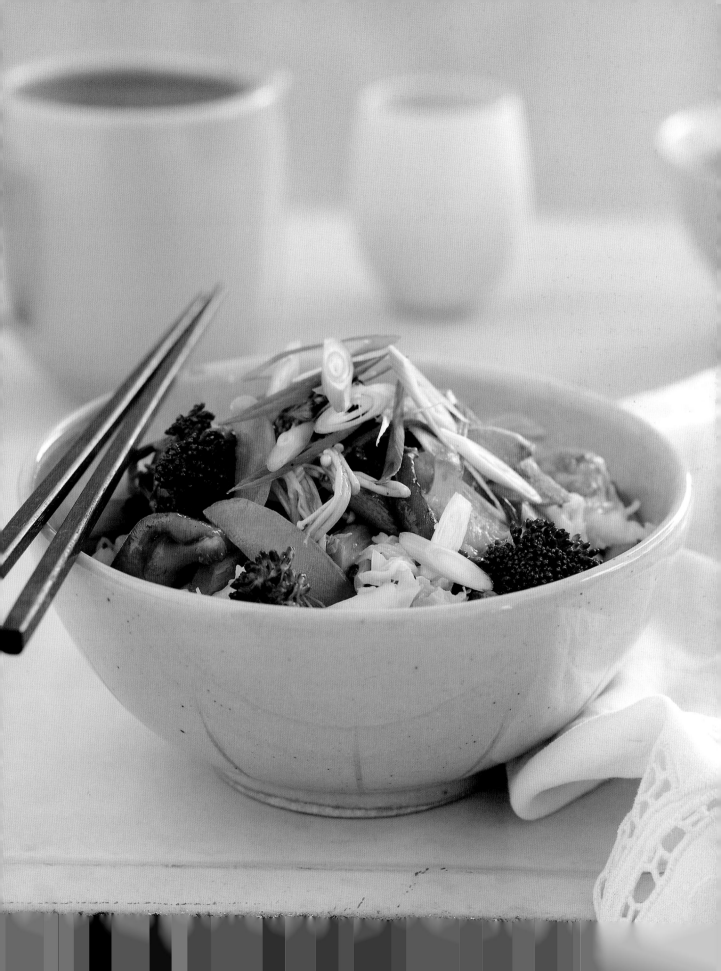

Zucchini, eggplant and mushroom lasagne

Serves 6
Prep 15 minutes
Cook 45 minutes
229 cal per serve

---

1 large eggplant, cut into 3 cm
  cubes
3 medium zucchini, thickly sliced
1 bunch English spinach, trimmed
2 cups low-cal ricotta
1 cup freshly chopped parsley
½ cup freshly chopped basil
2 garlic cloves, crushed
50 g grated parmesan
freshly ground black pepper
100 g mixed mushrooms, thinly
  sliced
3 large sheets fresh lasagne
½ cup salt-reduced chicken stock
4 handfuls salad leaves, to serve

I love reheated vegie lasagne, it always seems so much tastier. I've put this recipe together to make 6 serves. And don't panic about high-carb pasta meals – this is only 229 calories per serve!

Preheat oven to 190°C. Lightly grease a 32 cm × 20 cm ovenproof dish.

Place the eggplant in a steamer basket over simmering water. Steam for 8 minutes until tender. Remove and steam zucchini for 3 minutes. Remove and steam spinach for 1 minute until wilted and bright green. Drain spinach and coarsely chop.

Combine ricotta, herbs, spinach, garlic and half of the parmesan in a large bowl. Season to taste with pepper then set aside.

Spread ¼ of ricotta mixture over base of prepared baking dish. Top with a lasagne sheet and half of the vegetables. Repeat layering with lasagne, ricotta and remaining vegetables. Finish with a layer of lasagne and cover with remaining ricotta. Pour over stock and sprinkle with remaining parmesan.

Cover with foil and bake for 30 minutes. Preheat grill and remove foil. Place lasagne under grill, 10 cm away from heat, for 3–4 minutes, and grill until cheese is golden.

Serve with salad.

Tip

• Freeze any remaining lasagne sheets in batches of 3 for another use.

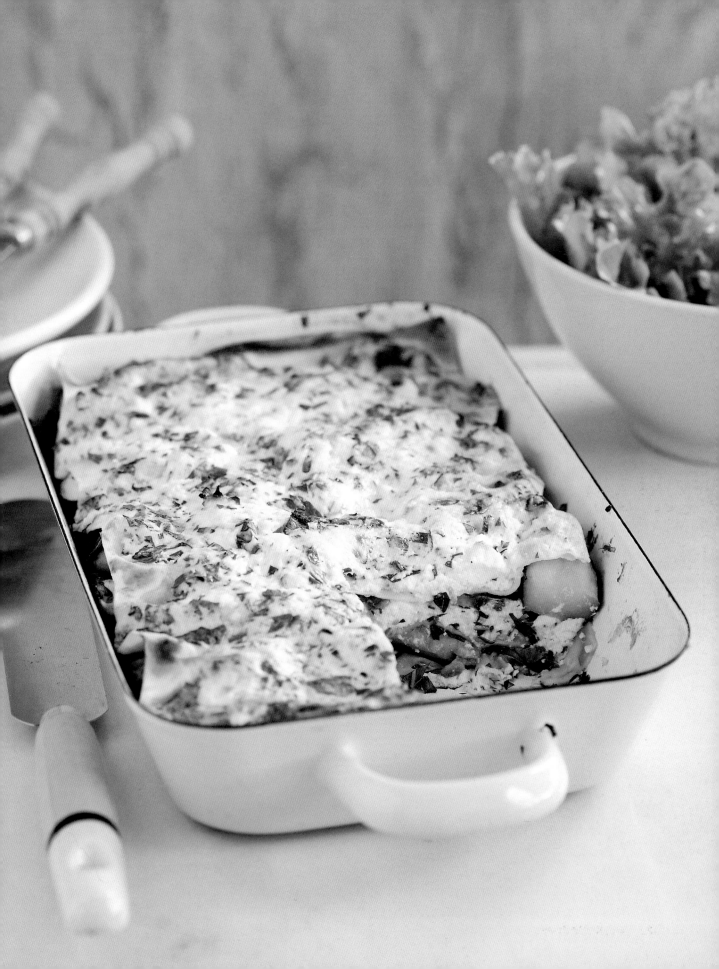

Cauliflower, spinach and ricotta bake

Serves 2
Prep 10 minutes
Cook 30 minutes
244 cal per serve

1 small cauliflower, broken
   into florets
1 bunch English spinach, trimmed,
   washed
3 teaspoons cornflour
1 cup skim milk
½ cup low-cal ricotta
pinch freshly grated nutmeg
freshly ground black pepper
2 tablespoons grated parmesan
4 handfuls salad leaves, to serve

Cauliflower is a seriously undervalued vegie that's jam-packed with vitamins, minerals and anti-cancer properties. Combining it with the folate-rich spinach in this recipe makes this one of the healthiest dishes in the book! Get into it!

Preheat oven to 220°C.

Place cauliflower in a steamer basket over simmering water and steam for 10 minutes until just tender. Remove, then steam spinach for 1 minute until wilted and bright green. Drain and coarsely chop.

Meanwhile, combine the cornflour and ¼ cup of milk in a jug. Place the remaining milk in a small saucepan and bring to the boil. Whisk in the cornflour mixture. Cook, stirring continuously, for 1 minute, until the sauce boils and thickens. Stir in the ricotta and nutmeg until smooth. Season with pepper.

Arrange the cauliflower and spinach in a single layer in a 24 cm × 17 cm ovenproof dish. Spoon the ricotta sauce over the vegies and then sprinkle with the parmesan. Bake for 20 minutes until the cheese is golden.

Serve with salad.

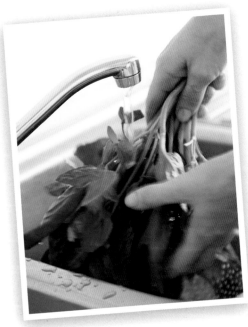

Tips
• Use a pinch of dried nutmeg if you don't have fresh.

Zucchini, green bean and mint risotto

Risotto is easy to cook and can be varied with lots of different ingredients, so it's a dish you'll want to have in your repertoire. It also comes under the heading of 'efficient' as it allows you to use up chicken stock or vegetable stock that you may have in the freezer. I tend not to eat a lot of risotto if I am trying to get into a pair of jeans that aren't zipping up easily. I don't usually have it for dinner, either, but it does make a great Sunday lunch before a long walk.

Place the stock and 2 cups water in a medium saucepan and bring to a simmer on medium heat.

Heat the olive oil in a large, heavy-based saucepan on medium heat, then add the onion and cook, stirring, for 5 minutes or until softened. Add the rice and stir to coat with the oil. Add a ladle of the simmering stock and cook over medium heat, stirring, until the stock has been absorbed. Continue for 10 minutes, adding another ladle of stock as each is absorbed, stirring constantly.

Add the zucchini and beans. Continue adding stock, a ladle at a time, stirring constantly, until the risotto is cooked, about another 10 minutes. Taste the rice – it should be soft but retain a bit of bite.

Remove from the heat. Stir in the parmesan and set aside, covered, for 5 minutes.

Stir through the mint and season to taste with pepper. Serve with the rocket.

Tips

• The risotto will still be quite 'saucy' when you remove the pot from the heat, but the rice will soak up the sauce as it rests.

• I like my vegies with a bit of crunch, but if you like them soft, add them 5 minutes earlier than I say in the method.

Serves 2
Prep 10 minutes
Cook 30 minutes
361 cal per serve

---

1 cup reduced-salt chicken
   or vegetable stock
1 tablespoon olive oil
1 onion, finely chopped
½ cup arborio rice
2 zucchini, cut into batons
100 g green beans, trimmed
   and cut into 3 cm lengths
¼ cup grated parmesan
2 tablespoons shredded mint
freshly ground black pepper
4 handfuls rocket, to serve

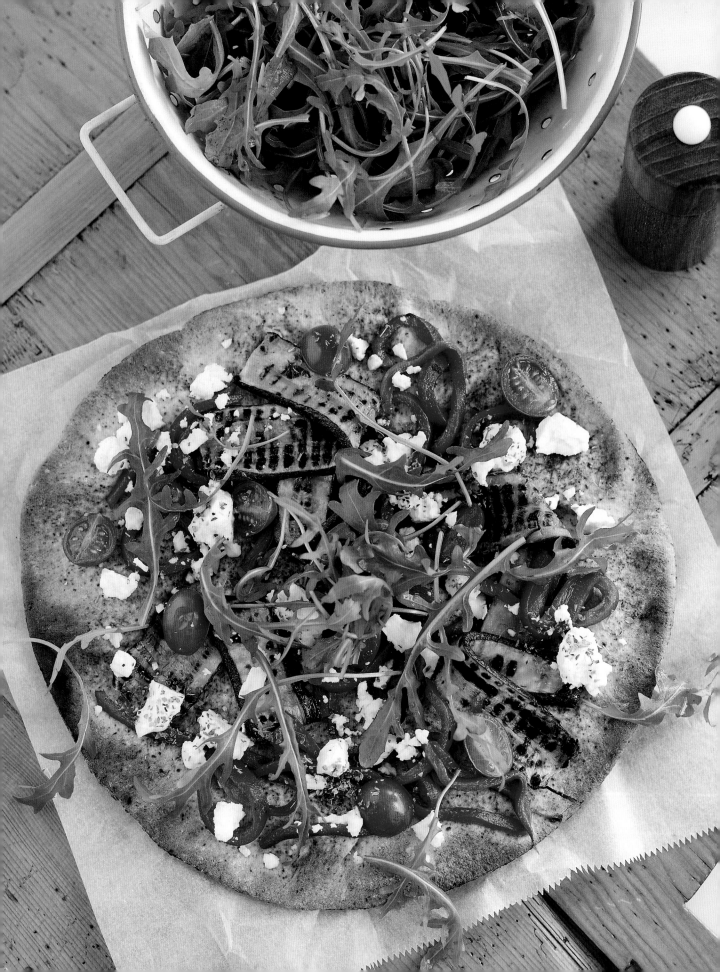

Grilled capsicum and zucchini pizza with feta

I never eat those crappy fast-food pizzas, as I believe they are partly responsible for the obesity crisis we're now facing. Plus they taste like cardboard. This one tastes great – and at just 10 minutes to prepare and cook, it's way quicker than a home delivery.

Preheat the grill to hot. Place the pita breads under the grill for 1 minute until crisp, then remove from the grill and rub the grilled side with the garlic. Turn each pita over and brush with olive oil. Top with capsicum, zucchini, tomato (cut-side up) and feta. Sprinkle with oregano and season with pepper.

Place under the grill for 2 minutes until the cheese lightly browns. Serve with the rocket.

Serves 2
Prep 5 minutes
Cook 5 minutes
314 cal per pizza

2 medium-sized wholemeal pita breads (23 cm in diameter)
1 garlic clove, halved
½ teaspoon olive oil
100 g char-grilled capsicum, cut into strips (see page 106)
100 g char-grilled zucchini strips (see page 106)
50 g roma cherry tomatoes, halved
50 g low-cal feta, crumbled
¼ teaspoon dried oregano
freshly ground black pepper
4 handfuls rocket, to serve

Wholemeal penne with zucchini, lemon zest and parsley

Serves 2
Prep 10 minutes
Cook 15 minutes
356 cal per serve

125 g wholemeal penne
1 zucchini, cut into batons
50 g sugarsnap peas, trimmed
½ lemon, zest and juice
1 garlic clove, crushed
¼ cup coarsely chopped parsley
1 tablespoon extra virgin olive oil
50 g low-cal ricotta

For me, this is a bit of a treat meal and I tend to have it for lunch rather than dinner as the calories are quite high. Try to get flat-leafed (Italian) parsley as it looks the best, and take care not to overcook the peas and zucchini. Oh, and if you can't get sugarsnap peas, try snowpeas.

Cook the penne in a large saucepan of boiling, salted water according to the packet directions. Add zucchini and peas 2 minutes before the end of the cooking time. Drain.

Toss through the lemon zest and juice, garlic, parsley and olive oil. Sprinkle over ricotta.

Tip
• Buy fresh ricotta from the deli section as packaged ricotta has a higher moisture content and can make your dish look a bit sloppy.

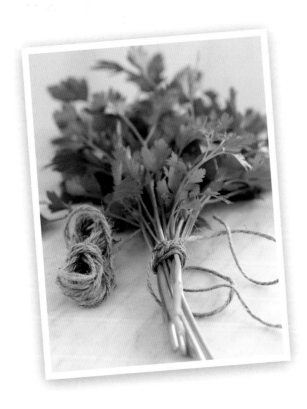

Lentil, leek and mushroom loaf

A great meal that ticks all the boxes: low-calorie, delicious, and perfect for more than one meal. Make it on the weekend, then pop a slice on a bed of lettuce in an airtight container and take it to work for lunch. I prefer to cook my own lentils, but to help you get used to the recipe I've given you the canned lentil version first up.

Preheat oven to 180°C. Lightly grease a 25 cm × 11 cm loaf pan.

Heat the oil in a frying pan on medium. Cook the leek and mushrooms for 10 minutes, stirring until softened. Transfer to a bowl. Add lentils, oats, ricotta, egg, lemon juice, parsley and curry powder. Season with pepper and mix until combined. Spoon the mixture into the greased loaf pan. Cook for 45 minutes. Allow to stand for 5 minutes before slicing with a serrated knife.

Serve with steamed squash.

Tip

• If you prefer to cook your own lentils rather than use canned ones, gently boil 1 cup of dried green or yellow lentils for 40 minutes until soft. Drain well and use as described above.

Serves 4
Prep 15 minutes
Cook 55 minutes
261 cal per serve

1 tablespoon olive oil
1 leek, finely chopped
150 g mixed mushrooms, finely chopped
2 × 400 g cans lentils, drained, rinsed, 1 can mashed with ¼ cup water
⅔ cup oats
¼ cup low-cal ricotta
1 egg
1 tablespoon lemon juice
½ cup freshly chopped parsley
1 teaspoon curry powder
freshly ground black pepper
400 g steamed squash, to serve

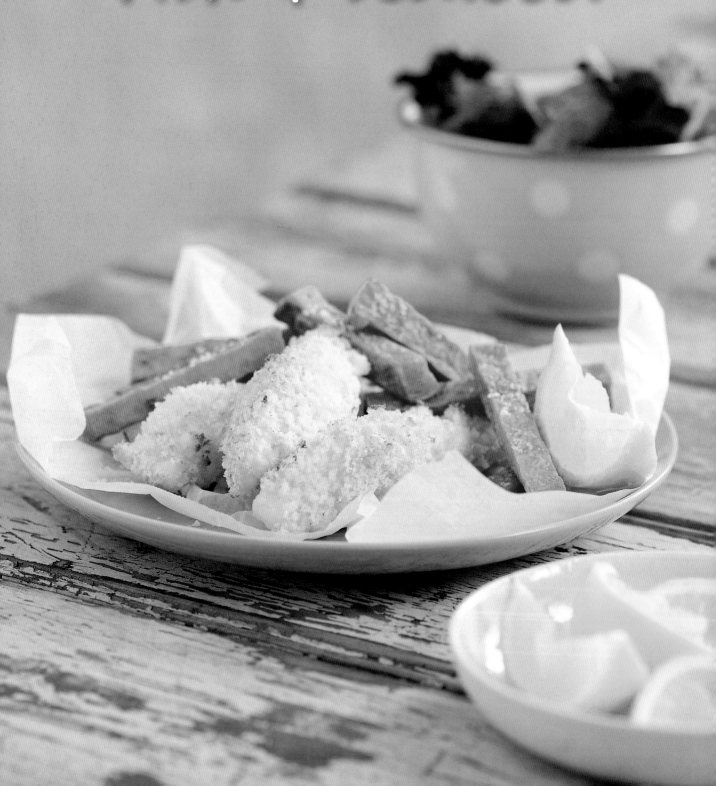

Fish & seafood

Baked fish and chips

Deep-fried battered fish and chips: taste? Greasy. Nutritional value? Questionable. After effects? You feel bloated and queasy. Oven-baked fish with sweet potato chips: taste, nutritional value and after-effects? Sensational!

Preheat the oven to 220°C. Line 2 baking trays with baking paper and lightly spray with oil.

Cut the sweet potato into 1.5 cm slices. Cut the slices into chips and place on the prepared tray. Spray lightly with oil and bake for 30 minutes, turning occasionally.

Meanwhile, cut the fish into 15 cm × 5 cm strips. Toss in flour, then dip in the egg and coat with breadcrumbs. Place on the second tray and put into the oven with the sweet potato. Bake the fish for 5–10 minutes, depending on thickness.

Serve the fish with the chips, lemon wedges and mixed leaves.

Variation

• Spice up this dish by adding herbs and spices to the breadcrumbs – try crushed dill seeds, fresh tarragon or fresh thyme.

Serves 2
Prep 15 minutes
Cook 40 minutes
362 cal per serve

olive oil spray
300 g sweet potato, peeled
250 g firm white fish fillets
1 tablespoon plain flour
1 small egg, lightly beaten
¼ cup fresh breadcrumbs (see page 139)
1 lemon, cut into wedges, to serve
2 large handfuls mixed salad leaves, to serve

Whole baked snapper with fennel, onion and tomato

Serves 4
Prep 10 minutes
Cook 45 minutes
328 cal per serve

2 large fennel bulbs, thinly sliced
2 onions, sliced
3 garlic cloves, thinly sliced
2 tablespoons olive oil
1 × 1.3 kg whole snapper, scaled
  and gutted
freshly ground black pepper
1 lemon, sliced
3 tomatoes, sliced
160 g mixed salad leaves, to serve

There is something special about getting a well-prepared meal out of the oven. I love the anticipation and the aroma as I open the oven door. This baked snapper recipe is really useful to have in your repertoire, as you can use the same principles to prepare other fish.

Preheat the oven to 220°C. Place the fennel, onion and garlic in a large baking dish (28 cm × 37 cm). Drizzle over half the olive oil and toss to coat. Roast for 15 minutes. Remove the dish from the oven.

Season the fish cavity with a sprinkle of pepper. Place half the lemon inside the cavity. Lay the fish over the vegetables and season. Top the fish with the remaining lemon slices and half the tomato, and drizzle over the remaining olive oil. Scatter the remaining tomato around the fish.

Roast for 30 minutes until the vegetables are tender and the fish is just cooked. Serve the fish and vegetables drizzled with pan juices, along with the salad leaves.

Tips
- Choose a nice fresh fish (the eyes should be clear and shiny).
- Use the fish bones and boil them up to make a stock for a soup.

Variations
- Try this recipe with salmon, trout, barramundi or bream.
- Try placing some herbs in with the lemon, such as parsley or rosemary.

Salmon patties with tomato salsa

These are a really good alternative to minced-beef burgers, and for my money taste ten times better. The salsa is dead easy to make and really turns this recipe into something special. My favourite tomatoes are ox-hearts – ask for them at your greengrocer.

Cook the sweet potato in a saucepan of boiling, lightly salted water for 10 minutes until tender. Drain, then return to the pan and place on a low heat for 1 minute until the sweet potato is thoroughly dry. Remove from the heat and mash lightly with a fork. Add the milk, beating until very smooth. Set aside to cool completely.

Flake the salmon into a bowl. Add the mashed sweet potato and shallots. Season to taste and mix well to combine. Divide into 6 patties. Dust with flour, brush with beaten egg and coat with breadcrumbs. Place on a tray and refrigerate for 1 hour.

To make the salsa, combine all the ingredients in a bowl.

Heat the olive oil in a large, non-stick frying pan on medium. Cook the patties for 4–5 minutes each side until golden. Serve with the tomato salsa and lemon wedges.

Tips

- Make sure you allow at least an hour to chill the patties; otherwise, they'll break up when you cook them.
- Put a few patties aside, or make a double quantity, to freeze for later – they will be a time saver on another day.

Serves 2
Prep 15 minutes
Cook 20 minutes
Chill 1 hour
339 cal per serve

250 g sweet potato, cut into chunks
2 tablespoons skim milk
210 g can pink salmon, drained
2 shallots, finely chopped
freshly ground black pepper
2 tablespoons plain flour
1 egg, lightly beaten
¼ cup fresh wholemeal breadcrumbs (see page 139)
3 teaspoons olive oil
lemon wedges, to serve

tomato salsa
2 tomatoes, diced
¼ small red onion, finely chopped
1 cup roughly chopped parsley

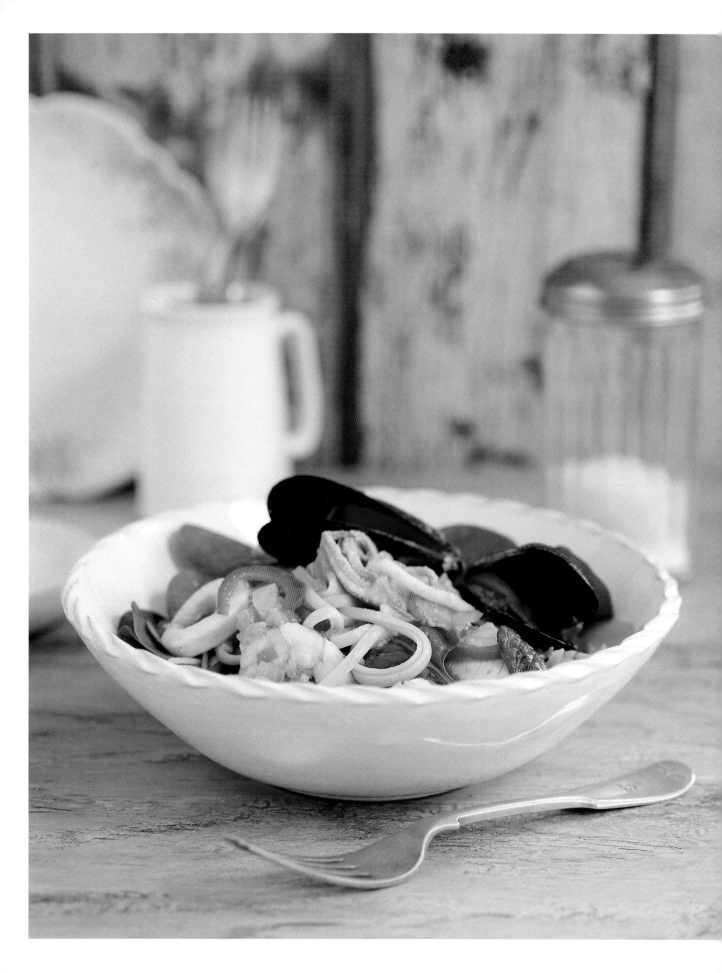

Seafood linguini

This is my husband's favourite pasta dish. To keep the calorie intake down for myself, I simply serve up more marinara, less linguini and more salad. Marinara mix is a cheaper way of buying delicious seafood, but try to buy it fresh, and make sure that your fishmonger gives you a good selection that includes fish, prawns, scallops and mussels (no crab sticks, thank you – they're highly processed and very salty).

Cook the pasta in a large saucepan of boiling, lightly salted water according to the packet directions. Drain, reserving ¼ cup cooking liquid.

Meanwhile, lightly spray a large, non-stick frying pan with oil and heat on high. Cook the marinara mix and garlic for 2–3 minutes, stirring, until cooked through. Remove from the pan and set aside.

Lightly spray the pan again with oil and heat on medium–high. Cook the onion and capsicum for 3 minutes, stirring, until softened. Add the tomato and reserved cooking liquid and cook, stirring, for 3 minutes until the sauce thickens. Reduce the heat to low.

Add the pasta to the pan and toss with the sauce until well coated. Stir through the spinach and half the marinara mix. Cook until the spinach wilts.

Serve the linguini and sauce topped with the remaining marinara mix.

Tip
- Add a pinch of salt to the water before boiling (but don't add oil – there's no reason to), and then prepare the seafood and sauce while the pasta is cooking.

Serves 2
Prep 10 minutes
Cook 15 minutes
377 cal per serve

100 g dried linguini pasta
olive oil spray
200 g marinara mix
3 garlic cloves, crushed
1 onion, chopped
1 red capsicum, cut into strips
2 tomatoes, diced
3 handfuls baby spinach

Tomato, anchovy and basil pizza

Makes 2
Prep 5 minutes
Cook 5 minutes
307 cal per pizza

2 medium-size wholemeal pita
  breads (23 cm in diameter)
1 garlic clove, halved
½ teaspoon olive oil
8 anchovy fillets, halved
150 g roma cherry tomatoes,
  halved
⅓ cup grated low-cal mozzarella
freshly ground black pepper
2 tablespoons small basil leaves
4 handfuls rocket, to serve

Kids are more likely to eat food they have cooked themselves, and pizza is a good meal for them to have fun making. This is one of my two favourite pizzas (the other is capsicum and zucchini pizza with feta; see page 127), and it has a real Mediterranean flavour. It's just 10 minutes to prepare and cook, and only around 300 calories per pizza. I find that if you get too heavy-handed with your ingredients, not only will the calories escalate, but the pizza will become a mess. Be disciplined with the cheese please. Less is best here.

Preheat the grill to hot. Place the pita breads under the grill for 1 minute until crisp. Remove from the grill and rub the grilled side with the garlic. Turn each pita over and brush with olive oil. Top with the anchovy slices and the tomato, cut-side down. Sprinkle with mozzarella and season with pepper.

Place under the grill for 2 minutes until the cheese has melted and started to brown. Scatter over the basil and serve with the rocket.

Variations

• Instead of anchovies, add 100 g char-grilled capsicum (see page 106) and ¼ cup small black olives (320 calories).
• Try 50 g cooked artichoke heart and 100 g smoked salmon. Serve with a drizzle of lemon juice (300 calories per pizza).

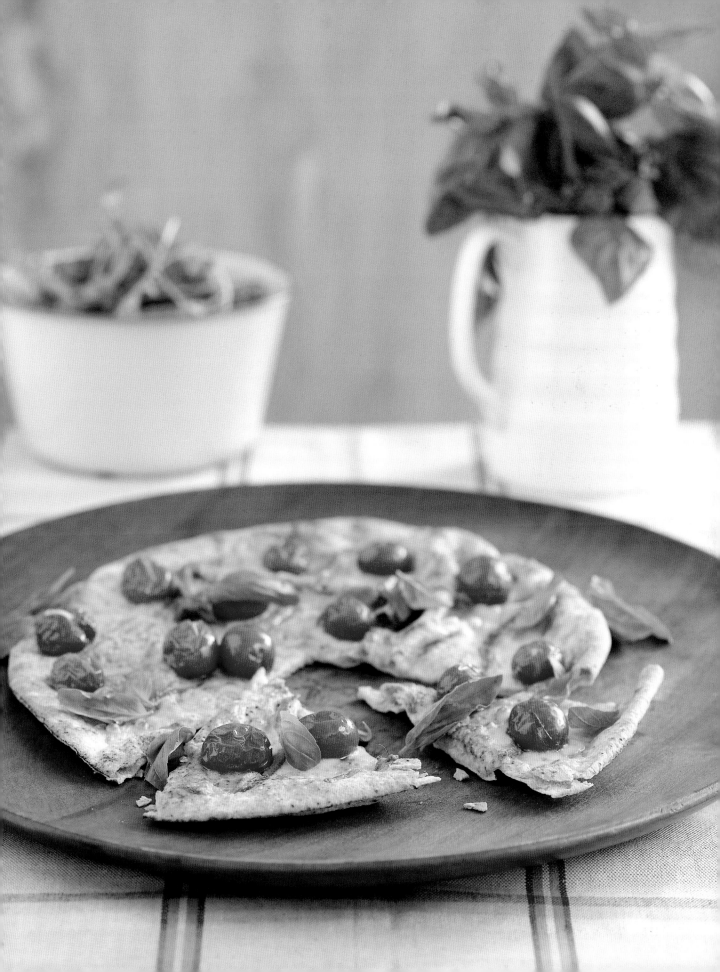

Chinese steamed trevalla with baby bok choy

Serves 2
Prep 10 minutes
Cook 10 minutes
233 cal per serve

25 g ginger, peeled and cut
   into thin strips
2 × 150 g skinless blue-eye
   trevalla fillets
3 shallots, shredded
2 bunches baby bok choy,
   trimmed
2 tablespoons soy sauce
1 teaspoon sesame oil
⅓ cup coriander leaves

Steamed fish would have to be one of the healthiest 'meat' dishes you can eat, but it can be bland if it's not prepared thoughtfully using herbs and spices. Lemon or lime juice and zest go hand in hand with steamed fish, too.

Scatter half the ginger in a steamer. Arrange the fish in the steamer and scatter with the shallots and remaining ginger. Place the baby bok choy to one side. Steam, covered, over a large frying pan of simmering water for 8–10 minutes or until cooked to your liking.

Meanwhile, heat the soy sauce and oil in a small saucepan on medium for 1 minute until hot. Drizzle the sauce over the fish and top with the ginger, shallots and coriander leaves. Serve with the steamed bok choy.

Tip

- If you don't have a steamer, wrap the fish, ginger, shallots and bok choy in baking paper and cook in a preheated oven at 200°C for 15 minutes.

Variation

- To create a Mediterranean-style variation, steam the fish over a handful of basil leaves and 2 sliced tomatoes and scatter with 2 teaspoons capers. Drizzle cooked fish with 1 teaspoon extra-virgin olive oil and scatter over 2 tablespoons black olives and extra basil leaves. Serve with 4 handfuls salad leaves (210 calories per serve).

Tuna mornay

I grew up with tuna mornay, and it's still a yummy meal that doesn't have to be heavy on the calories, providing you don't go overboard with the cheese. Use ramekins for serving as they help you control portion sizes.

Preheat the oven to 200°C. Drain the tuna, reserving 1 tablespoon of the springwater, then flake the tuna.

Combine the cornflour and ¼ cup milk in a jug. Place the remaining milk in a medium saucepan and bring to the boil. Whisk in the cornflour mixture. Cook, stirring, for 1 minute until the sauce boils and thickens. Stir in 2 tablespoons of the cheese, and the tuna, peas and corn, shallots, lemon juice and reserved tuna water. Season with pepper.

Spoon the tuna mixture into a 3-cup ovenproof dish or 2 × 1½ cup ramekins. Combine the remaining cheese with the breadcrumbs and sprinkle over the tuna mixture. Bake for 20 minutes until golden and bubbly. Serve with the salad leaves.

Serves 2
Prep 5 minutes
Cook 25 minutes
317 cal per serve

180 g can tuna in springwater
3 teaspoons cornflour
¾ cup skim milk
⅓ cup grated low-cal tasty cheese
2½ cups frozen peas and corn
2 shallots, finely chopped
1½ tablespoons lemon juice
freshly ground black pepper
1 tablespoon fresh breadcrumbs
4 handfuls salad leaves, to serve

Tips

- Tuna mornay freezes really well, so why not double the recipe and freeze the extra in individual ramekins.
- To make your own **breadcrumbs**, leave a few slices of bread out to dry (loosely covered with a clean tea towel). Process in a blender or place in a plastic bag and crush with a rolling pin. You can also toast the slices in a low oven (150°C) until crisp. Cool to room temperature before processing or crushing. Store them in an airtight container, or freeze if you've made a big batch so they won't go stale. It's a bit of effort, but they taste so much better than packaged ones.

Stir-fried snapper with shallots, broccolini and shiitake mushrooms

Serves 2
Prep 15 minutes
Cook 10 minutes
335 cal per serve

300 g snapper fillet, skinned
    and cut into cubes
2 garlic cloves, crushed
1 tablespoon freshly grated ginger
2 tablespoons salt-reduced soy
    sauce
1 tablespoon olive oil
1 bunch broccolini, stems
    quartered lengthways, cut
    into chunks
2 yellow zucchini, halved
    lengthways and sliced
6 shallots, cut into 5 cm pieces
150 g shiitake mushrooms, sliced

I particularly like this dish as it includes my favourite stir-fry ingredients – broccolini, shiitake mushrooms and ginger. Fish stir-fries really well and because it's mixed with strong flavours in this recipe you don't have to shell out for a more exotic fish species to enjoy the taste. The less expensive choices are often more environmentally responsible, too – try bream, flathead or whiting as alternatives.

Combine the fish, garlic, ginger and 1 tablespoon of the soy sauce in a bowl. Set aside.

Heat 2 teaspoons of the olive oil in a wok on high. Stir-fry the broccolini for 3 minutes. Add the zucchini and stir-fry for another 2 minutes. Remove from the wok.

Heat 1 teaspoon of the remaining oil and stir-fry the shallots and mushrooms for 2 minutes until the onions soften. Remove from the wok.

Heat the remaining oil and stir-fry the fish for 2 minutes until browned. Return the vegetables to the wok with the remaining soy sauce and toss to coat.

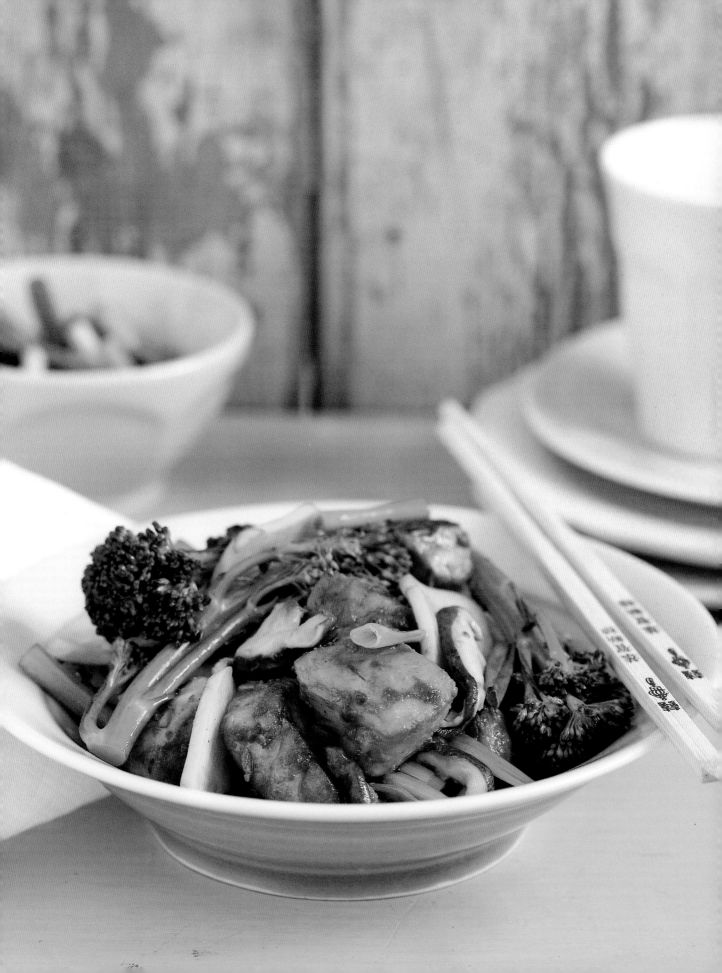

Tuna kebabs

Serves 2
Prep 15 minutes
Cook 5 minutes
319 cal per serve

zest and juice of ½ lemon
1 garlic clove, crushed
280 g fresh tuna, cut into 3 cm
    cubes
400 g can artichoke hearts,
    drained and halved
1 yellow capsicum, cut into 3 cm
    cubes
12 black olives, pitted
freshly ground black pepper
100 g cherry tomatoes (preferably
    truss)
4 handfuls rocket, to serve

Why would you barbecue a rotten old sausage when you could toss a couple of these little beauties on the barbie? Try and get the truss variety of cherry tomatoes if you can, and leave the stalks on them – it gives the dish a great Mediterranean feel.

If using wooden skewers, soak them in water for 30 minutes. Combine the lemon zest and juice with the garlic in a small bowl and set aside.

Thread the tuna, artichoke hearts, capsicum and olives alternately onto 4 large (or 6 smaller) skewers and place in a shallow dish. Just before cooking, season the kebabs well with pepper and pour over the lemon mixture, turning to coat well.

Lightly spray a char-grill pan with oil and heat on medium. Cook the kebabs for 3–4 minutes, turning regularly, until lightly charred and cooked through. Meanwhile, cook the tomatoes on the same char-grill for 4 minutes until lightly charred and warm. Serve the kebabs with the grilled tomatoes and the rocket.

Barbecued ginger and lemon prawns

Serves 2
Prep 15 minutes
Marinate 10 minutes
Cook 5 minutes
195 cal per serve

500 g large uncooked prawns,
    peeled and deveined, tails intact
1 tablespoon freshly grated ginger
1 garlic clove, crushed
freshly ground black pepper
olive oil spray
2 tablespoons lemon juice
½ cup coriander leaves
750 g Asian greens (e.g. bok choy,
    Chinese cabbage, gai larn),
    steamed, to serve

I find it's easy to get stuck in the same old barbecuing habits, and an Asian influence is a nice change. This ginger (spicy!) prawn recipe is one of my favourites. You don't need to marinate the prawns for long – around 10 minutes is enough to infuse them with flavour. Just 2 or 3 minutes is enough time to cook them through.

Combine the prawns, ginger and garlic in a bowl. Season with pepper. Marinate for 10 minutes.

Preheat a barbecue hot plate or heavy frying pan on high and lightly spray with oil. Just before cooking, add half the lemon juice to the prawns and toss to coat. Cook the prawns for 2–3 minutes until they are pink and cooked through. Drizzle over the remaining lemon juice and transfer to a serving plate. Top with the coriander and serve with the steamed greens.

Spicy stir-fried prawns with snowpeas, asparagus and wombok

Wombok is Chinese cabbage, and it has a fabulous sweet flavour – so sweet, in fact, that you can use it instead of lettuce in sang choy bow (see page 157). It keeps really well in the fridge – pop it in the crisper and it'll be good for a couple of weeks. This is another one of my 'staple' recipes – get clever with it, then tinker with the ingredients to suit what you have in the fridge.

Combine the prawns, shallots, chilli, garlic and half the soy sauce in a bowl.

Heat the oil in a wok on high. Stir-fry the prawn mixture in 2 batches for 2 minutes until the prawns are pink. Remove from the wok. Add the snowpeas, asparagus and ¼ cup water and stir-fry for 3 minutes until just tender and the water has evaporated. Return the prawns to the wok with the wombok and the remaining soy sauce. Stir-fry for 2 minutes until the wombok just wilts. Serve immediately.

Variation

- Replace the prawns with octopus (343 calories per serve), calamari (276 calories) or marinara mix (353 calories).

Serves 2
Prep 20 minutes
Cook 10 minutes
291 cal per serve

500 g medium uncooked prawns, peeled and deveined
3 shallots, finely chopped
1 long red chilli, finely chopped
2 garlic cloves, crushed
2 tablespoons salt-reduced soy sauce
1 teaspoon vegetable oil
150 g snowpeas, trimmed
1 bunch asparagus, trimmed and cut into chunks
250 g wombok (Chinese cabbage), coarsely shredded

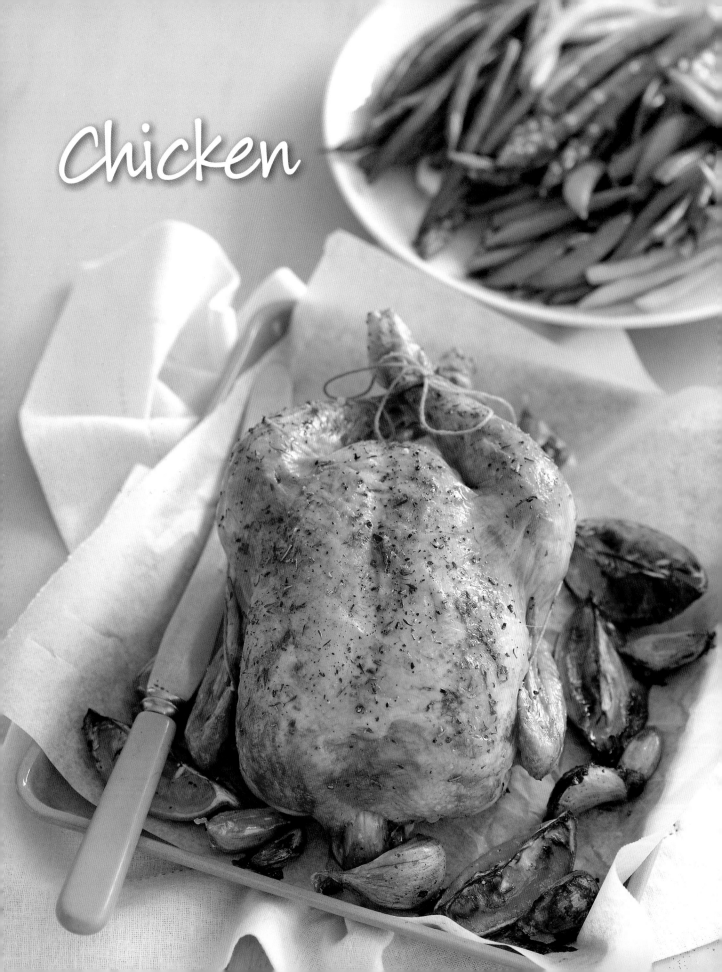

Chicken

Roast lemon and oregano chicken with mixed vegetables

Guests always feel special when a whole roast chicken has been cooked in their honour. Suddenly everyone remembers the Sunday roasts of their childhood, and the way the aroma used to fill the house. Steer clear of the skin – it bumps up the calories to 416 per serve.

Preheat the oven to 200°C. Pat the chicken dry with paper towel. Halve 1 lemon and cut the other lemon into quarters. Squeeze ½ lemon into the chicken cavity, then place the squeezed fruit inside. Sprinkle in half the oregano and season with pepper. Truss the chicken with kitchen string so that it cooks evenly – tie the wings so they are held close to the body, and cross the ends of the drumsticks together and tie with several loops of string.

Lightly spray the chicken with cooking oil. Season to taste with pepper and sprinkle over the remaining oregano.

Place the chicken on a rack in a baking dish and scatter around the garlic cloves and lemon quarters. Roast for 50 minutes, basting regularly. Squeeze the remaining ½ lemon over the chicken. Roast for another 10 minutes, or until the chicken juices run clear when you pierce the thickest part with a skewer. Stand, loosely covered, for 5 minutes before carving.

Meanwhile, steam the vegetables in 2 batches in a large vegetable steamer for 3 minutes until just tender. Drain and toss with the olive oil in a warm dish. Season to taste with pepper. Serve the chicken with the mixed vegetables.

Tip
- Remember that this serves 6, so place any leftovers in the fridge for making sandwiches or taking for lunches.

Serves 6
Prep 15 minutes
Cook 1 hour
339 cal per serve

1 × size 17 chicken, trimmed and washed
2 lemons
1 tablespoon dried oregano
freshly ground black pepper
olive oil spray
1 head garlic, broken into cloves
200 g green beans, trimmed
200 g yellow beans, trimmed
200 g snowpeas, trimmed
200 g sugarsnap peas, trimmed
2 bunches asparagus, trimmed and halved
1 tablespoon extra virgin olive oil

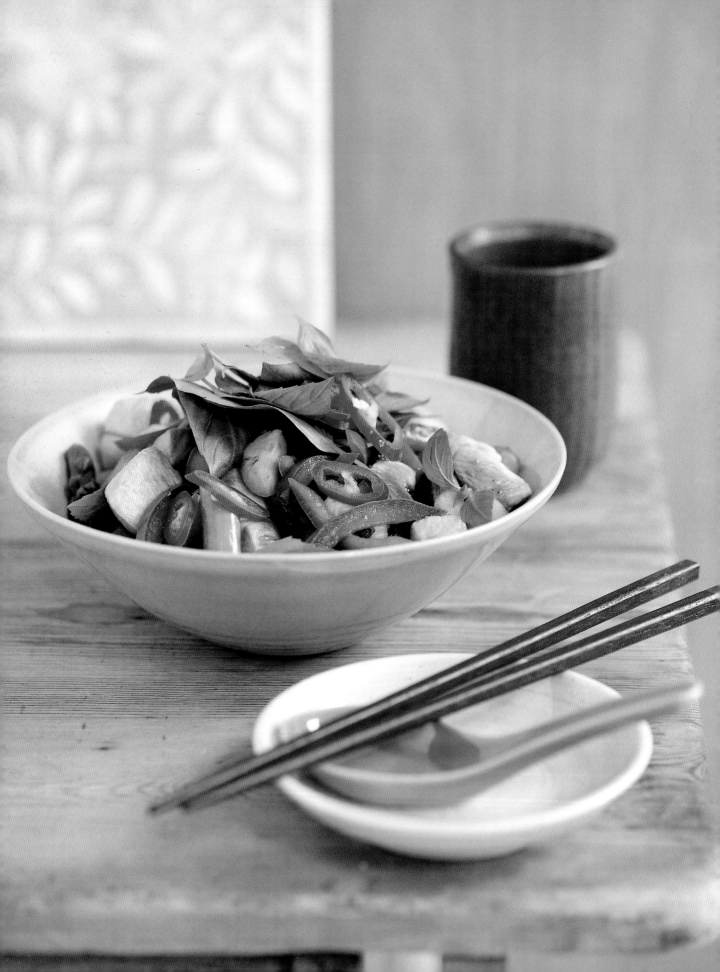

Thai chicken stir-fry

This stir-fry is an excellent choice if you're serious about losing weight. The water chestnuts are low in calories and salt and provide a great texture contrast. Thai basil is beautifully aromatic, but don't fret if you can't get it – just use ordinary basil.

Heat 1 teaspoon of the oil in a wok on high. Stir-fry the chicken in 2 batches for 2 minutes until browned and cooked through. Set aside.

Heat the remaining oil in the wok. Add the asparagus, capsicum, water chestnuts and half the basil. Stir-fry for 3–4 minutes until the asparagus and capsicum are just tender. Return the chicken to the wok with the fish sauce and toss to coat.

Transfer to a serving bowl and scatter with the chilli and remaining basil to serve.

Tips

- If you can find fresh water chestnuts, they taste much better than the canned variety. Wash them well and peel with a sharp knife, removing any bruises. To prevent them going brown, place each water chestnut into cold water after peeling.
- To feed the family serve with brown, basmati or doongara rice.

Serves 2
Prep 15 minutes
Cook 10 minutes
315 cal per serve

2 teaspoons vegetable oil
300 g chicken breast fillet, trimmed and cut into 1.5 cm cubes
1 bunch asparagus, cut into chunks
1 green capsicum, thinly sliced
227 g can whole water chestnuts, drained, rinsed and halved
1 cup torn Thai basil leaves
3 teaspoons fish sauce
1 long red chilli, thinly sliced on the diagonal

Spicy Cajun chicken kebabs with mixed leaf salad

Serves 2
Prep 15 minutes
Cook 15 minutes
286 cal per serve

---

300 g sweet potato, peeled and thickly sliced
220 g chicken breast fillet, trimmed and cut into 2 cm cubes
2 teaspoons Cajun seasoning
1 green capsicum, cut into 2 cm cubes
¼ red onion, cut into 2 cm pieces
olive oil spray
4 handfuls mixed lettuce leaves, to serve
1 lemon, cut into wedges, to serve

Kebabs are fantastic. Not only are they delicious and fun to prepare, but having to pull them apart means you slow down the eating process and feel fuller. Cajun seasoning can be bought ready made or you can make your own (see below). This is another meal to get the kids involved in – they love threading the kebabs!

If using wooden skewers, soak 6 skewers in water for 30 minutes before threading on the chicken and vegetables.

Cut each slice of sweet potato into quarters. Place the sweet potato in a microwave-safe bowl and microwave on high for 3 minutes or until just tender. Combine the chicken and Cajun seasoning in a bowl. Toss to coat. Thread the chicken, sweet potato, capsicum and red onion alternately onto skewers.

Lightly spray a char-grill pan with oil and heat on medium. Cook the kebabs for 10–12 minutes, turning regularly, until lightly charred and the chicken is cooked through. Serve the chicken kebabs (3 skewers per person) with the salad leaves and lemon wedges.

Tips

• Make sure you cut all the vegies and chicken the same size so that they cook evenly.

• If you don't have a microwave, steam the sweet potato in a vegetable steamer for about 8 minutes over simmering water. Don't boil the water, or the sweet potato will be too watery.

• To make your own **Cajun seasoning**, cook 1 teaspoon each cumin, coriander and fennel seeds in a small frying pan on low heat for 2 minutes, stirring. Grind finely using a pestle and mortar. Mix with 1 teaspoon each of paprika, mustard powder, onion powder and ground oregano, ¼ teaspoon garlic powder and a tiny pinch of cayenne pepper. Store in an airtight container.

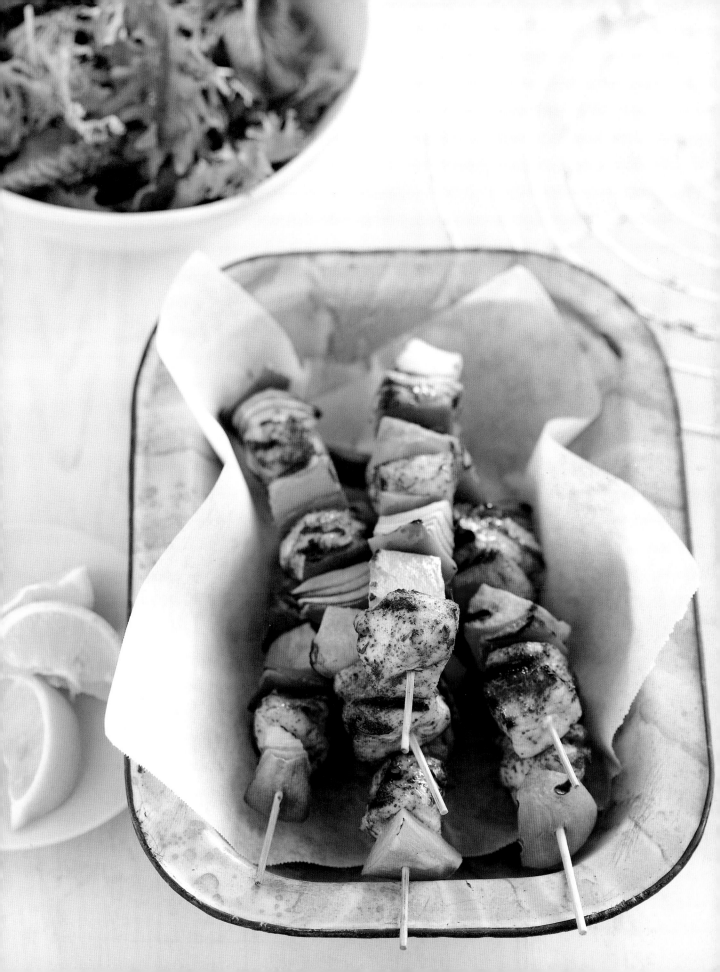

Thai green chicken curry

Serves 2
Prep 15 minutes
Cook 15 minutes
368 cal per serve

---

1 tablespoon green curry paste
1 cup light coconut-flavoured
    evaporated milk
2 baby eggplants, thickly sliced
1 large carrot, cut into batons
150 g green beans, trimmed
    and halved
1 bunch asparagus, trimmed
    and cut into chunks
200 g chicken breast fillet,
    trimmed and thinly sliced
1 tablespoon lime juice
1 teaspoon fish sauce
¼ cup Thai basil leaves, to serve

Everyone knows that green curries are calorie central, but mine is an unbelievable 368 calories per serve. With the extra vegies and delicious sauce, you won't even notice that there's no rice. This is a treat meal I might have on a Saturday night after having done a two-hour session that morning – it's not something I have regularly.

Heat the curry paste in a large saucepan on medium heat for 30 seconds until fragrant. Stir in the evaporated milk. Add the eggplant, carrot, beans and asparagus. Gently simmer for 8 minutes until just tender. Remove the vegetables with a slotted spoon and keep warm. Add the chicken, lime juice and fish sauce to the pan. Cook, stirring, for 3 minutes until the chicken is cooked through. Return the vegetables to the pan and gently toss to coat.

Serve the curry scattered with the basil leaves.

Tips
- Slice the eggplant just before adding to the dish; otherwise, it will oxidise and go brown.
- If you can't get Thai basil, just use ordinary basil.
- If you're feeding the troops, just adjust the quantities and boil up some basmati or brown rice to serve with it.

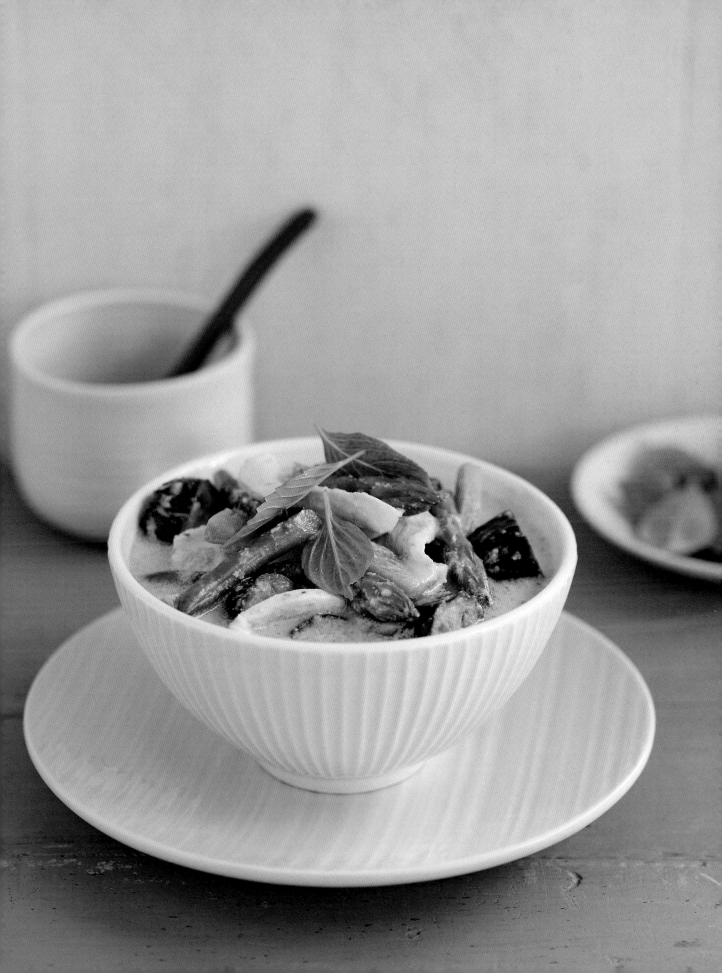

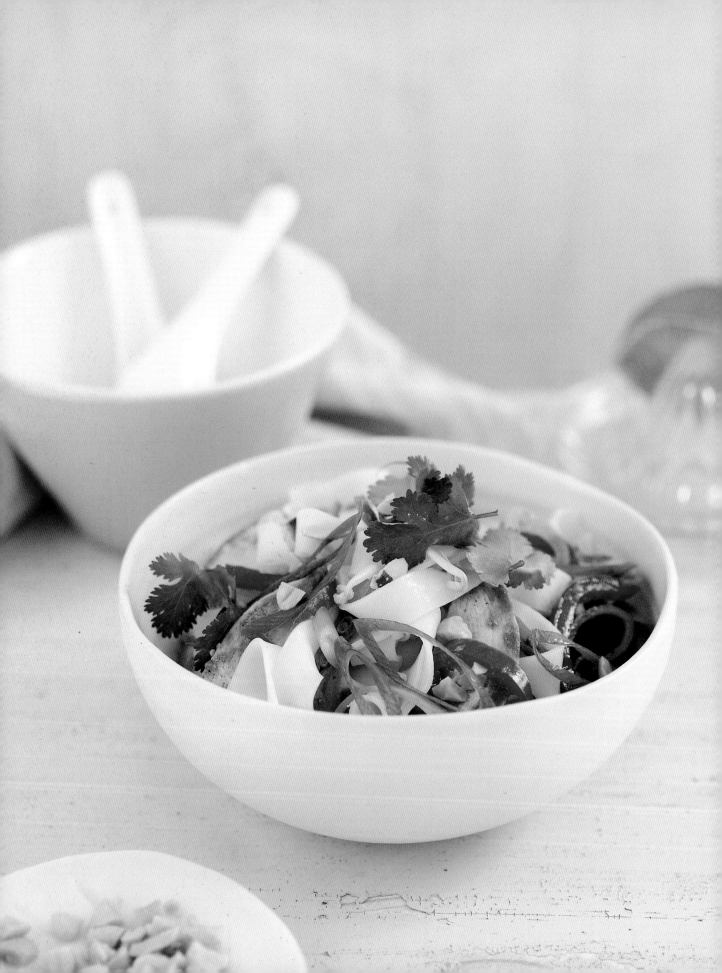

Chicken pad thai

I never eat this dish in restaurants because its fat content is *off the scale*, but I love my version because I've taken out all the calories and left in all the flavour. Don't be afraid of the long list of ingredients. You can always vary the vegies, as long as you keep the sauce recipe exactly the same and watch out for the peanuts! This is another special-occasion meal, not a regular one for me.

Soak the rice noodles in hot water for 20 minutes until softened. Drain well.

Meanwhile, lightly spray a large non-stick wok with oil and heat on medium–high. Stir-fry the chicken for 2–3 minutes until browned and cooked through. Set aside. Lightly spray the wok again and stir-fry the onion for 1 minute. Add the capsicum and snowpeas and stir-fry for another 4 minutes until just tender. Add the garlic and stir-fry for 30 seconds.

Return the chicken to the wok, then add the noodles, fish sauce, lime juice and palm sugar. Toss gently to combine. Remove from the heat. Toss through the bean sprouts, shallot and coriander.

Garnish with the peanuts and serve with lime wedges.

Tips

- Soaked noodles tend to break, so don't toss them for too long.
- Stick to 1 tablespoon of chopped peanuts, otherwise you'll turn this meal into a calorie-fest!

Variation

- Try using other vegies, such as baby corn instead of snowpeas, or use half and half.

Serves 2
Prep 20 minutes
Cook 20 minutes
344 cal per serve

---

100 g dried rice-stick noodles
olive oil spray
150 g chicken breast fillet, trimmed and thinly sliced
1 small onion, halved and thinly sliced
1 red capsicum, thinly sliced
150 g snowpeas, thinly sliced on the diagonal
2 garlic cloves, crushed
1 tablespoon fish sauce
1 tablespoon lime juice, plus lime wedges to serve
2 teaspoons grated palm sugar
1 cup bean sprouts
1 shallot, sliced on the diagonal
½ cup freshly chopped coriander leaves
1 tablespoon chopped peanuts, toasted, to serve

Char-grilled chicken with tomato salsa

Serves 2
Prep 10 minutes
Cook 15 minutes
321 cal per serve

olive oil spray
220 g chicken breast fillet,
   trimmed

tomato salsa
1 large corn cob
2 tomatoes, diced
1 Lebanese cucumber, diced
125 g can four-bean mix,
   drained and rinsed
½ cup coarsely chopped coriander
2 teaspoons lemon juice
1 garlic clove, crushed

Fast, tasty, low in calories and high in nutrition, this dish is a classic in my kitchen. Hear me loud and clear on this one: if you can cook a tasty chicken breast you will equip yourself with one of the best resources available to manage your weight. I sometimes take out the beans in this recipe to decrease the calories and I *always* cook extra chicken to use for sandwiches or salads.

Lightly spray a char-grill pan with cooking oil and heat on medium–high. Cook the corn for 14 minutes, turning regularly, until lightly charred and tender. Meanwhile, on the same char-grill cook the chicken for 8–10 minutes each side until lightly charred and cooked through. Cover and rest the chicken for 2 minutes before slicing.

To make the salsa, cut the corn kernels off the cob and combine them with the remaining ingredients.

Serve the chicken alongside the salsa.

Variations

- If you prefer to grill your chook, pop it on a cast-iron skillet, give it an olive oil spray and grill it for 5 minutes each side.
- I like to slice a 'pocket' in the side of the breast and stuff it with herbs, such as rosemary and thyme, before cooking.
- You can bring the calories down even further by making the salsa without the beans; it's just as yummy, but only 284 calories per serve.

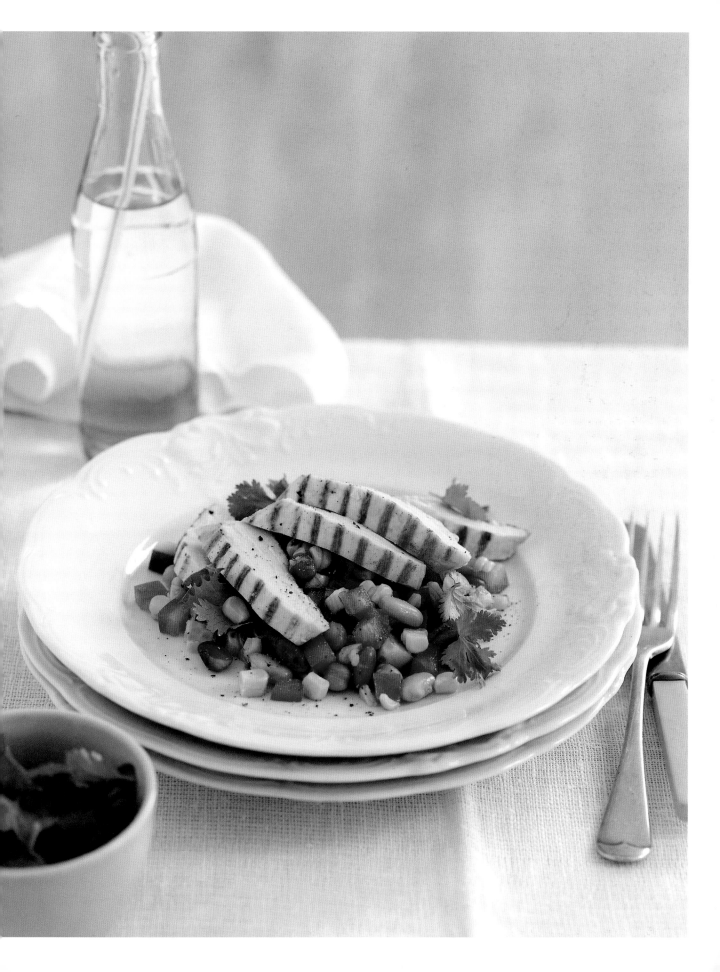

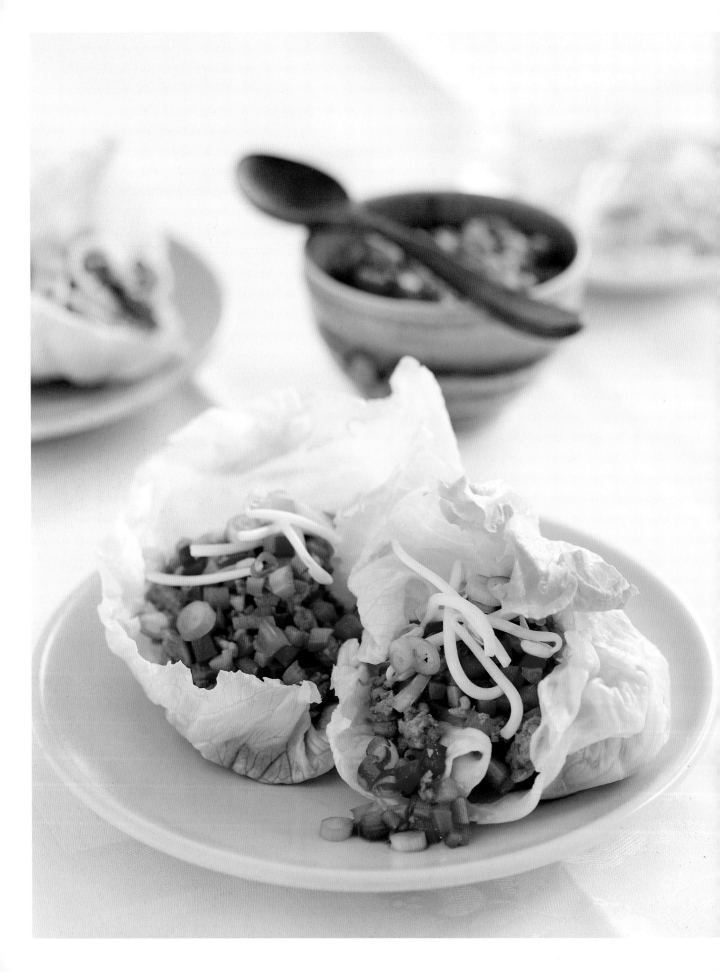

Chicken sang choy bow

This is a great family meal – fun to prepare and delicious to eat. The kids will love it because it's so hands-on. The more you can get them involved, the better – they're more likely to tuck into something they've helped to prepare.

Select the best lettuce leaves and if necessary trim them with scissors to make at least 6 large 'cups'. Place in a large bowl filled with iced water to crisp.

Lightly spray a wok with oil and heat on high. Stir-fry the chicken and half the shallots for 2 minutes until the chicken is cooked through. Add the carrot, celery, capsicum, sauces and garlic. Stir-fry for another 4 minutes. Transfer immediately to a serving bowl. Scatter with the remaining shallots.

To serve, arrange the lettuce cups on a platter with the bean sprouts. Spoon a little chicken mixture into each leaf, top with several bean sprouts and fold the lettuce over to enclose the filling. Eat with your hands.

Tip

- To feed a family of four, simply double all quantities of chicken, vegetables and sauces.

Serves 2
Prep 15 minutes
Cook 10 minutes
248 cal per serve

1 large iceberg lettuce
olive oil spray
220 g lean chicken mince
2 shallots, finely sliced
1 medium carrot, diced
2 celery stalks, diced
1 red capsicum, diced
3 teaspoons hoisin sauce
2 teaspoons salt-reduced
  soy sauce
1 garlic clove, crushed
2 handfuls bean sprouts

Mediterranean chicken parcels

Serves 2
Prep 20 minutes
Cook 20 minutes
316 cal per serve

2 × 110 g chicken breast fillets, trimmed
olive oil spray
2 medium zucchini, sliced on the diagonal
200 g cherry tomatoes, halved
1 red capsicum, thinly sliced
1 garlic clove, thinly sliced
2 tablespoons fresh thyme
freshly ground black pepper
4 handfuls salad leaves
300 g can chickpeas, drained and rinsed
¼ red onion, halved and thinly sliced
2 teaspoons balsamic vinegar

These taste as spectacular as they look, and are not nearly as hard to make as you might think. You'll just need some baking paper and foil and a bit of patience.

Preheat the oven to 200°C. Pat the chicken dry with paper towel. Lightly spray a non-stick frying pan with oil and heat on medium. Cook the chicken for 1–2 minutes each side until browned.

Lay a chicken breast on one half of a large piece of baking paper. Top with half the zucchini, tomato, capsicum, garlic and thyme. Season to taste with pepper. Fold the paper over the chicken and wrap loosely, sealing the edges by folding and then pleating. Repeat with the other chicken breast and the remaining zucchini, tomato, capsicum, garlic and thyme. Wrap the parcels in foil if the paper isn't sealed completely. Lay the parcels on a baking tray and bake for 15 minutes.

Combine the salad leaves, chickpeas, red onion and vinegar in a bowl. Place the parcels on individual serving plates for everyone to open their own, and let your guests help themselves to salad.

Variations

• Try this recipe with skinless white fish fillets instead of chicken. The calorie count will drop to around 273 calories per serve. Depending on the thickness of the fillet, the fish should take around 10 minutes to cook.

• If you prefer to use dried chickpeas, cook ½ cup according to the packet directions and use as described above. You'll need to be organised, though. Soaking overnight is easier (see page 200) otherwise you'll have to boil them for an hour or more.

Chicken rice paper rolls

Like sang choy bow (see page 157), this is a great family meal to share around a big table. Kids love making their own rolls, which is great practice in taking responsibility for their own food. I've given you quantities to serve 2, but it's easy to adjust them to feed 4 or more.

Cook the noodles in boiling water for 2 minutes until tender, then drain well. Cool under cold water and drain again. Combine in a bowl with the chicken, carrot, bean sprouts and shallot.

One at a time, soak the rice paper sheets in room-temperature water for 30 seconds until soft. Lift out and place on a clean towel to absorb any excess moisture. For each rice paper sheet, place about 2 tablespoons of the vermicelli mixture on the lower half. Fold up the paper at the bottom, then fold the left and right sides over the filling. Add 2 large mint leaves and then roll up, pressing firmly to seal. Cover with a damp tea towel to prevent the roll from drying out. Repeat with the remaining rice paper and filling. Serve with sweet chilli sauce (optional).

Tip
- Drop the sweet chilli sauce if you are trying to lose weight.

Variations
- Instead of chicken try using 150 g peeled, cooked prawns (345 calories per serve) or 150 g smoked tofu (315 calories per serve).
- Leave out the chicken and make it a vegetarian dish (278 calories).

Serves 2 (6 rolls)
Prep 20 minutes
Cook 5 minutes
333 cal per serve (including sweet chilli sauce)

¼ × 250 g packet rice vermicelli noodles
80 g shredded cooked chicken
1 carrot, coarsely grated
½ cup bean sprouts, tails removed
1 shallot, finely chopped
6 round rice paper sheets (22 cm in diameter)
12 large mint leaves
2 tablespoons sweet chilli sauce (optional)

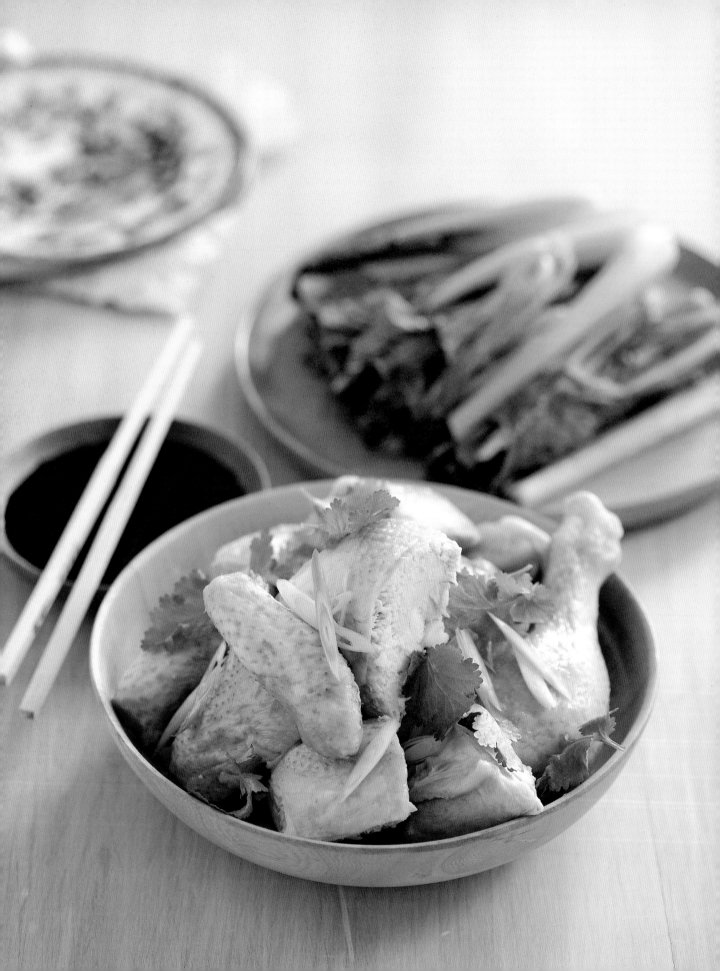

Chinese poached chicken

Seriously, this recipe changed my life! The chicken can be served hot or cold, but either way it is *sooooo* succulent and juicy. I love to make subtle changes to the flavour by introducing different herbs and spices to the water, and it makes fantastic stock.

Remove any visible fat from the chicken and pat dry with paper towel. Place breast-side down in a large, heavy-based saucepan. Add ⅔ of the shallots, all the ginger and half the salt. Add enough boiling water to just cover the chicken and bring to the boil on medium heat. Reduce the heat to low, cover and simmer for 10 minutes. Leaving the lid on, remove the pan from the heat and set aside for 45 minutes to finish cooking.

Remove the chicken from the pan and drain well over a large pan or bowl, particularly any liquid from the cavity. Strain the cooking liquid and any liquid collected from draining the chicken, and use as stock in other recipes.

Have ready a large bowl half-filled with cold water and ice cubes. As soon as the chicken is drained, carefully plunge it into the bowl of iced water. Leave for 15 minutes or until cold. Lift out carefully, drain thoroughly and pat dry with paper towel.

Place the chicken on a plate and rub all over with the sesame oil. Cover loosely with foil and refrigerate until ready to serve. Using a heavy knife, cut the chicken into pieces. Cut the remaining shallots into long, thin shreds. Toss the shallots with the coriander leaves and scatter over the chicken.

Place the choy sum in a steamer over simmering water and steam for 5 minutes until just tender. Serve the chicken with the steamed vegetables and soy sauce, if using.

Serves 6
Prep 20 minutes
Stand 1 hour
Cook 10 minutes
268 cal per serve

1 × size 15 chicken
6 shallots, cut into 8 cm lengths
30 g ginger, sliced
1 teaspoon salt
3 litres (about 12 cups) boiling water
2 teaspoons sesame oil
½ cup coriander leaves
3 bunches choy sum
soy sauce, to serve (optional)

Tips
- Don't be surprised when the chicken flesh has a slight pearly pink colour and the bones are a little red in the centre – it means the chicken is succulent and moist.
- Refrigerate any leftover portions for another meal, or for sandwiches.

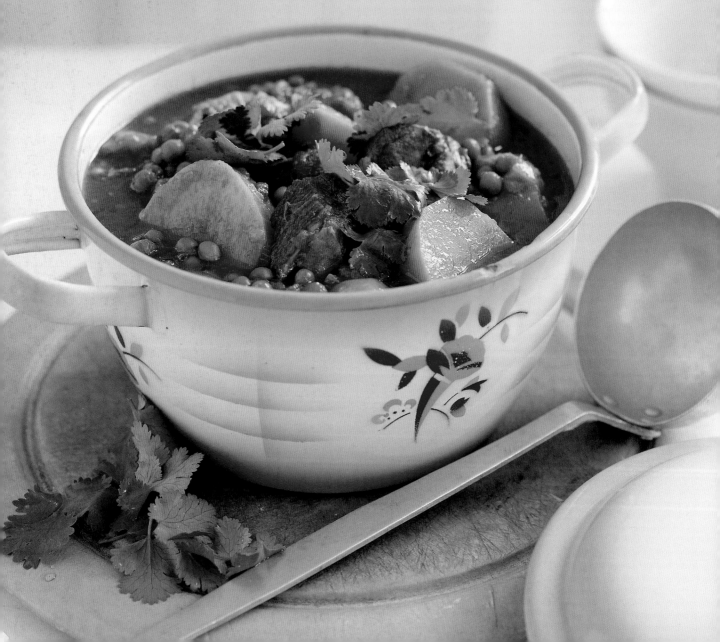

Lamb, beef & kangaroo

Lamb and sweet potato tagine

Once this lovely dish is prepared, it simmers on the stove for an hour, so you can get heaps of things done while it cooks. It's also a perfect meal for leftovers, saving you time on a weeknight. See page 97 for how to make your own Moroccan seasoning.

Serves 6
Prep 15 minutes
Cook 1¼ hours
296 cal per serve

Lightly spray a heavy-based casserole dish with oil and heat on medium–high. Cook the lamb in 2 batches for 3 minutes, turning regularly, until well browned all over. Set aside.

Heat the olive oil in the same dish. Cook the onion for 5 minutes, stirring, until softened. Stir in the garlic, ginger and seasoning. Cook for 30 seconds until fragrant. Return the lamb to the pan and toss well to coat. Add the tomato and ⅔ cup water. Bring to the boil. Reduce the heat and simmer, covered, for 1 hour.

Add the sweet potato and simmer, covered, for another 30 minutes. Add the peas and cook for another 3 minutes.

Just before serving, stir through the lemon juice. Sprinkle with the coriander to serve.

olive oil spray
650 g lamb shoulder, trimmed and cut into 4 cm cubes
2 teaspoons olive oil
1 onion, chopped
3 garlic cloves, crushed
1 tablespoon freshly grated ginger
1½ tablespoons Moroccan seasoning (see page 97)
400 g can diced tomatoes
850 g sweet potato, peeled and cut into 2 cm slices
1½ cups frozen peas
1 lemon, juice only
1 bunch coriander, leaves only, to serve

Tip
- Freeze individual servings of tagine for future use.

Variation
- Cook 1½ cups frozen broad beans separately in lightly salted boiling water for 2 minutes, drain and cool. Remove and discard the skins. Add the beans with or instead of the frozen peas.

Lamb shanks with green beans and mushrooms

Serves 6
Prep 15 minutes
Cook 1 hour 40 minutes
329 cal per serve

olive oil spray
6 lamb shanks, trimmed
2 teaspoons olive oil
1 onion, chopped
1 carrot, diced
1 large celery stick, diced
3 garlic cloves, crushed
½ cup red wine
1 cup salt-reduced beef stock
3 sprigs thyme
1 lemon, zest only
400 g button or Swiss brown
    mushrooms, halved or
    quartered depending on size
500 g green beans, trimmed

What a beautiful winter weekend dish to serve up to your friends or family. The lemon zest gives it a wonderful flavour (thank you, Margaret Fulton!). This dish tastes even better the next day, so making extra and refrigerating or freezing it is highly recommended.

Lightly spray a heavy-based casserole dish with oil and heat on medium–high. Cook the shanks in 2 batches for 3 minutes, turning occasionally, until well browned all over. Set aside.

Heat the olive oil in the same dish. Cook the onion, carrot and celery for 5 minutes, stirring, until softened. Stir in the garlic and cook for 30 seconds until fragrant. Return the shanks to the pan with the red wine and bring to the boil. Add the stock, thyme and lemon zest. Return to the boil, then reduce the heat to low and simmer, covered, for 1 hour, stirring occasionally so the shanks cook evenly. Add the mushrooms and simmer, covered, for another 30 minutes until the meat falls off the bone.

Meanwhile, cook the beans in a medium saucepan of boiling, lightly salted water for 8 minutes until tender. Drain. Stir the beans through the lamb stew when ready to serve.

Tips
- Don't worry if the shanks are not totally covered by the sauce when cooking. You don't want to dilute the sauce.
- Freeze individual servings for future use. Note that when this dish is refrigerated or frozen, any fat will rise to the top. Scrape it off before reheating.

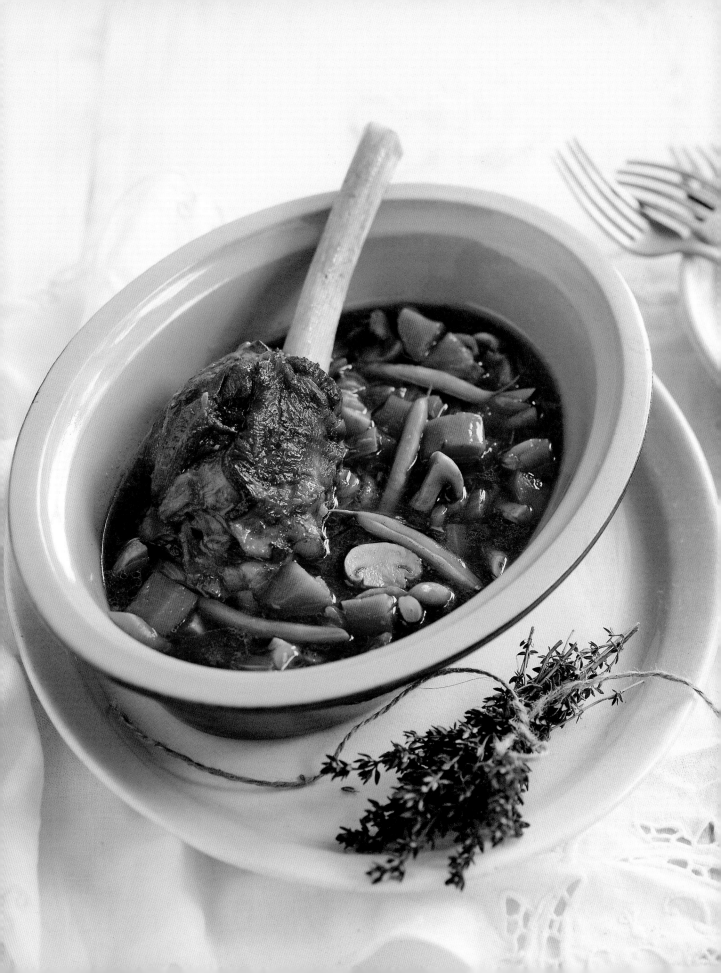

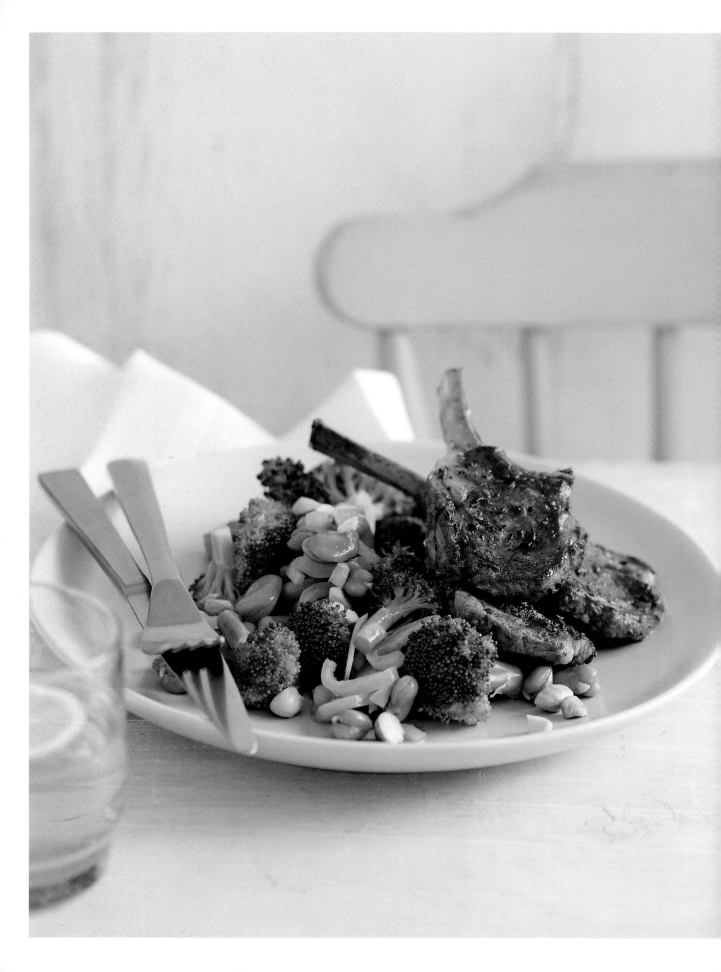

Cumin-crusted lamb cutlets with lemony broccoli and broad beans

I've served this one up a couple of times to lots of 'oohs' and 'ahs'. Make sure your butcher removes the fat from the cutlets, or do it yourself. A sprinkle of roasted almonds makes a lovely garnish for this meal, but don't worry if you don't have them.

Serves 2
Prep 10 minutes
Cook 15 minutes
321 cal per serve

1 cup frozen broad beans
1 large head of broccoli, broken into florets
6 lean lamb cutlets, ends trimmed of fat ('Frenched')
1 teaspoon cumin seeds, coarsely ground
freshly ground black pepper
olive oil spray
1 yellow banana chilli, seeded and sliced
1 garlic clove, thinly sliced
1 tablespoon lemon juice
1 tablespoon chopped roasted almonds (optional)

Cook the broad beans in a small saucepan of boiling, lightly salted water for 2 minutes. Remove the beans with a slotted spoon and cool in iced water. Drain. In the same pan of boiling water, cook the broccoli for 2 minutes until bright green. Drain and cool under cold water. Remove and discard the white broad-bean skins.

Coat the lamb cutlets with the cumin and season to taste with pepper. Lightly spray a non-stick frying pan with olive oil and heat on medium–high. Cook the cutlets for 2–3 minutes until browned and slightly pink inside. Remove from the pan and keep warm.

Wipe the pan clean and lightly spray with oil. Heat on medium. Cook the chilli and garlic for 2 minutes, stirring. Add the broccoli and beans and cook for another 2 minutes. Add the lemon juice, season with pepper and toss to coat.

Serve the broccoli and beans sprinkled with the almonds, if using, and alongside the lamb cutlets.

Variation

• You can cook the cutlets as a rack: pop them in a 200°C oven for 15-20 minutes for medium-rare, or 25-30 minutes for well done.

Open beef burgers

Serves 2
Prep 10 minutes
Cook 10 minutes
256 cal per burger

---

200 g lean beef mince
1 shallot, finely chopped
1 tablespoon low-cal barbecue
    sauce (optional)
freshly ground black pepper
olive oil spray
1 wholemeal bread bun, halved
    and hollowed out
4 iceberg lettuce leaves, shredded
80 g canned sliced beetroot
1 tomato, sliced
coarsely chopped parsley,
    to garnish

A real family-pleaser! Get your kids involved so they learn how to make a burger that won't give anyone a heart attack – they'll love being part of the cooking process. To lower the calories even further, I cut the buns in half and hollow out the middles so I can fill them up with salad, but you don't need to do that for husbands or growing children – they'll need a whole bun each.

Combine the beef mince, shallot and barbecue sauce (if using) in a bowl. Season to taste with pepper. With wet hands, shape the mixture into 2 patties.

Lightly spray a non-stick frying pan with olive oil and heat on medium. Cook the patties for 5 minutes each side until browned and cooked through.

Toast the bun halves, then line each bun with lettuce. Top with beetroot, a patty and tomato. Garnish with parsley and season with pepper.

Tips

• If you use a whole bread bun per person, the calorie count jumps to 342 per burger – almost 100 calories more!
• To lower your calories, flick the sauce and instead spice up your patties with a few slivers of chopped, fresh chilli.

Variation

• Sometimes I like to boil or steam fresh beetroot rather than use the canned variety, as it is crunchier and has a better flavour. But it does take a bit of time and can be messy. Small beetroots will take about 30 minutes to cook, while medium or large ones might take 1 hour or more. Wearing disposable gloves, rub the skins off the hot cooked beetroots under running water. Cool the beetroots a little before slicing.

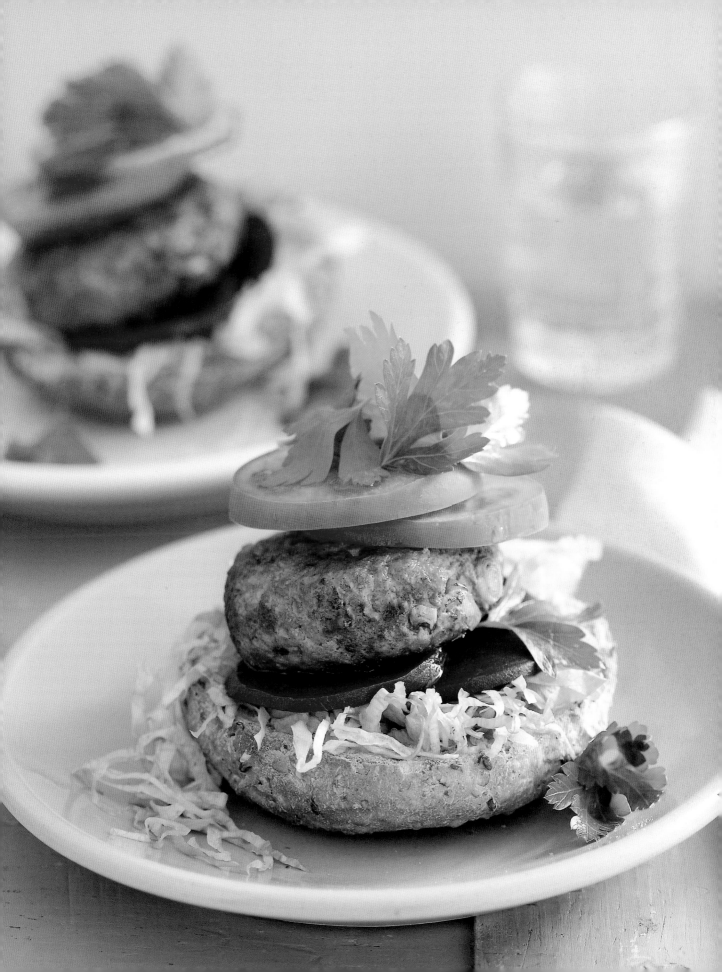

Spaghetti bolognese

Serves 2
Prep 15 minutes
Cook 35 minutes
422 cal per serve

125 g spaghetti
2 tablespoons shaved parmesan

bolognese sauce
olive oil spray
1 onion, finely chopped
2 garlic cloves, crushed
2 carrots, diced
1 zucchini, diced
1 celery stick, diced
100 g lean beef mince
400 g can diced tomatoes
2 tablespoons finely chopped
  parsley
1 teaspoon dried oregano

I bet you never expected me to include *this* stalwart in a calorie-conscious cookbook! My version has more vegies and fewer calories and is completely family friendly. I've given you ingredients for serving 2 people, but you'll easily adjust quantities for serving the hungry mob. This is brilliant for freezing and reusing for other meals.

To make the bolognese sauce, lightly spray a frying pan with olive oil and heat on medium. Cook the onion and garlic, stirring, for 5 minutes until softened. Add the carrot, zucchini and celery and cook, covered, for another 5 minutes, stirring occasionally.

Increase the heat to high. Add the mince and cook for 1 minute, stirring to break up any lumps, or until it has changed colour. Stir in the tomato, parsley, oregano and ½ cup water and simmer, covered, for 25 minutes, stirring occasionally.

Meanwhile, cook the spaghetti in a large saucepan of boiling, lightly salted water according to the packet directions. Drain.

Divide ⅔ of the bolognese sauce between 2 plates. Top with the spaghetti and the remaining sauce. Garnish with the parmesan.

Variations

• Serve the bolognese sauce with steamed bok choy if you are trying to lose weight (around 184 calories).

• I love using bolognese sauce as a base for **chilli con carne**. Just thaw 2 serves of the sauce, place in a pan, add a 400 g can of kidney beans (drained and washed) and ¼ teaspoon of chilli flakes or chilli powder and heat through. This will be around 300 calories per serve.

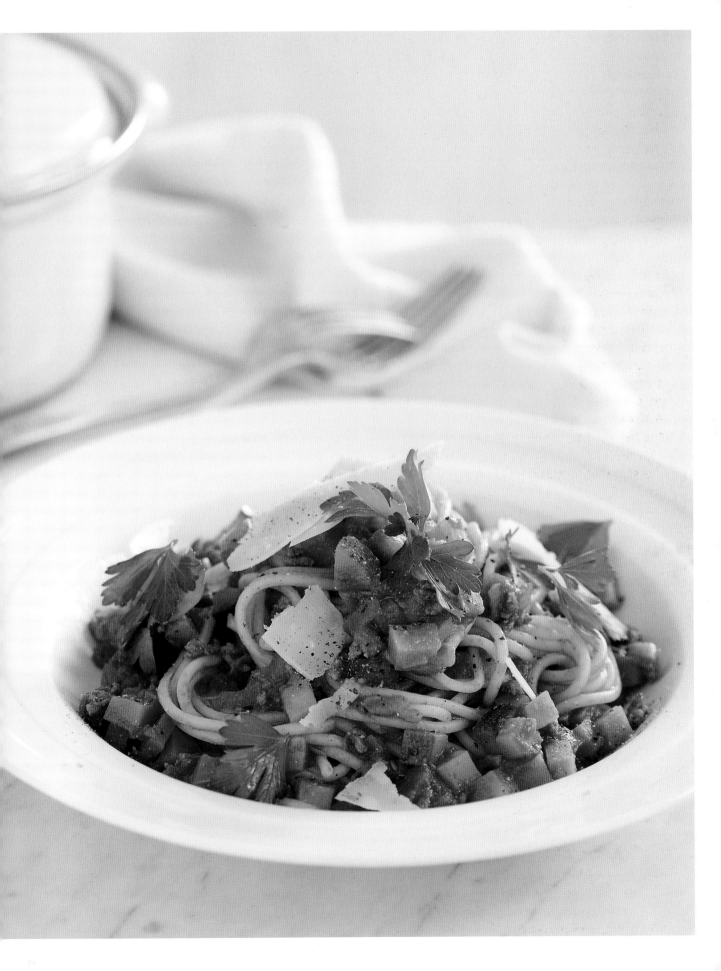

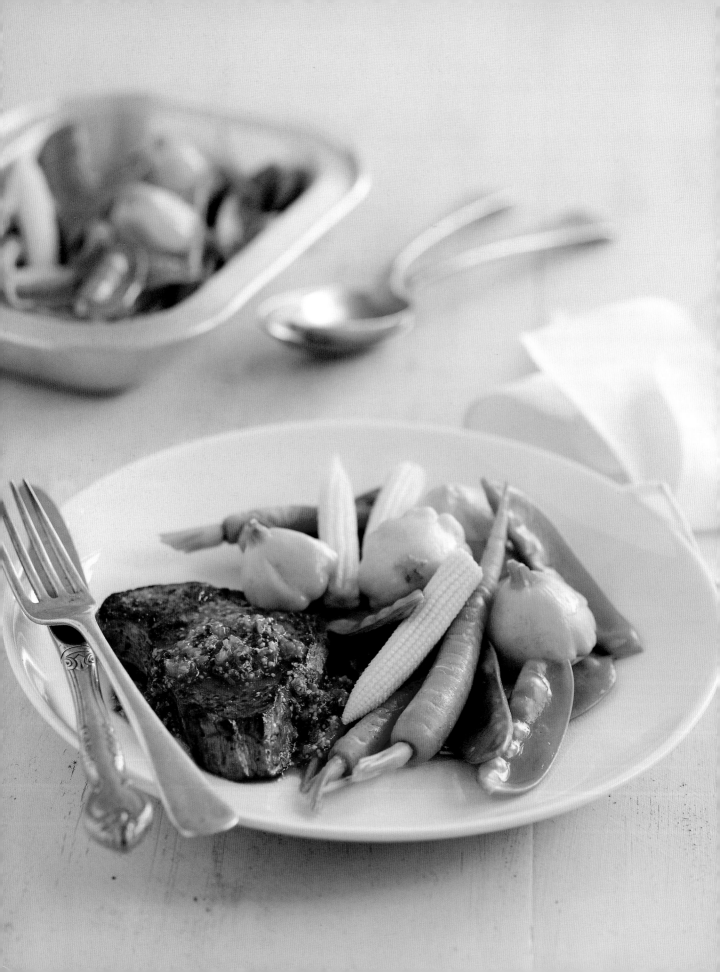

Mustard steak with steamed vegies

This mustard sauce is amazing, and will amp up even the cheapest cut of meat. The Dutch carrots and baby corn are delightfully sweet to balance the bite of the mustard.

Serves 2
Prep 15 minutes
Cook 15 minutes
313 cal per serve

Place the corn, squash and carrots in a steamer over a saucepan of boiling water. Steam for 5 minutes. Add the snowpeas and steam for another 3 minutes until just tender.

Meanwhile, lightly spray a large frying pan with olive oil and heat on high. Season the steaks with pepper and cook for 1–2 minutes each side for rare and 3–4 minutes for medium, depending on the thickness. Remove from the pan, cover and let stand for 3 minutes.

Meanwhile, reduce the heat to medium and cook the shallots in the frying pan for 2 minutes, stirring. Increase the heat and add the mustard, stock and ¼ cup water. Bring to the boil and simmer for 1 minute until thickened. Remove from the heat. Season to taste with pepper and stir in the parsley.

Drizzle the steak with mustard sauce and serve with the steamed vegetables.

115 g baby corn
6 yellow squash
½ bunch Dutch carrots, trimmed
150 g snowpeas, trimmed
olive oil spray
2 × 110 g rump steaks, trimmed
freshly ground black pepper

mustard sauce
1 shallot, finely chopped
3 teaspoons wholegrain mustard
¼ cup (60 ml) salt-reduced beef or chicken stock
2 tablespoons freshly chopped parsley

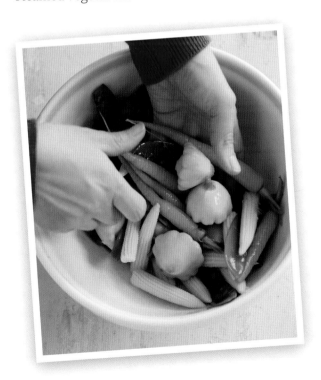

Spicy beef and vegetable meatloaf

Serves 6
Prep 15 minutes
Cook 1 hour
265 cal per serve

---

800 g lean beef mince
1 onion, finely chopped
1 large carrot, coarsely grated
1 zucchini, coarsely grated
½ cup rolled oats
5 tablespoons low-cal tomato
    sauce
2 tablespoons finely chopped
    parsley
1 tablespoon finely chopped
    thyme
2 garlic cloves, crushed
½ teaspoon salt
½–1 teaspoon chilli flakes
    (optional)
freshly ground black pepper
120 g mixed salad leaves, to serve

The preparation time on this is pretty quick but it has a long cooking time, so I prefer to cook it on the weekend. I often double the quantities, serving one lot to guests and slicing up the other to put in the fridge or freezer for other meals, which saves me time and money.

Preheat the oven to 180°C. Lightly grease an 11 cm × 25 cm loaf pan (6-cup capacity).

In a large bowl, combine the beef, onion, carrot, zucchini, oats, tomato sauce, herbs, garlic, salt, chilli (if using) and a good grinding of pepper. Knead the mixture with your hands until combined, then pack lightly into the prepared pan. Place on a baking tray and cook for 1 hour or until the loaf shrinks away slightly from the sides of the pan. Pour off any excess juices, then leave to stand for 10 minutes. Slice using a serrated knife and serve with the salad leaves.

Tips

- Leave the chilli out if you've cooking this one for kids.
- Wrap in individual portions to freeze for future lunches.

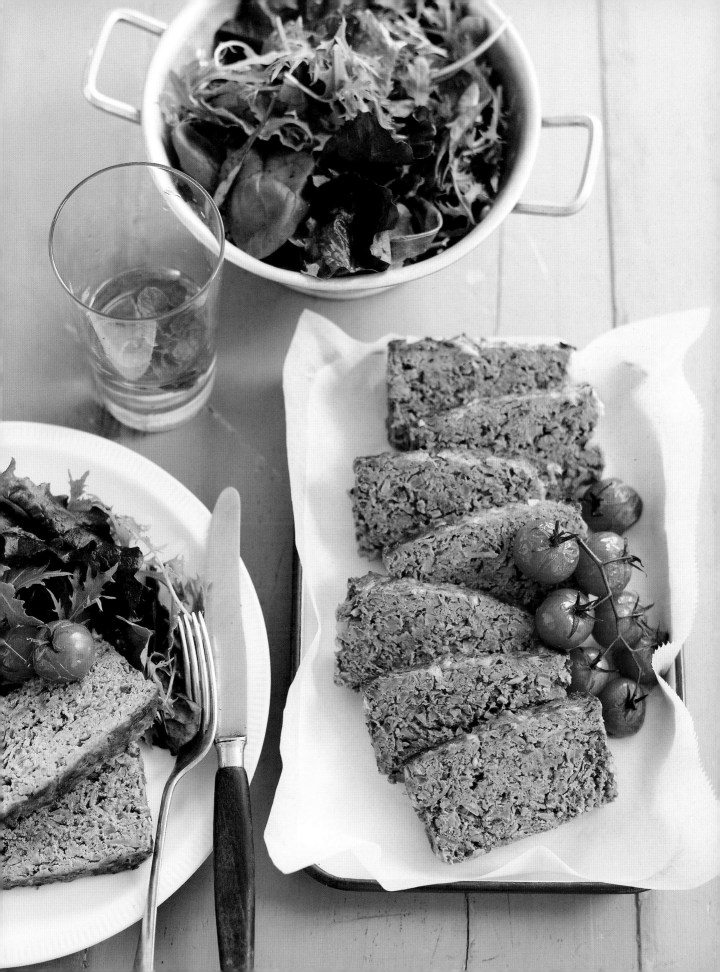

Zucchini, green bean and beef stir-fry with hoisin sauce

Serves 2
Prep 10 minutes
Cook 10 minutes
300 cal per serve

2 teaspoons vegetable oil
220 g rump steak, trimmed
 and cut into strips
200 g green beans, trimmed
 and halved
2 medium zucchini, halved
 lengthways and sliced on
 the diagonal
2 garlic cloves, crushed
2 teaspoons freshly grated ginger
1 tablespoon salt-reduced soy
 sauce
1 tablespoon hoisin sauce
1 bunch gai larn (Chinese
 broccoli), trimmed

If there's one meal that you need to be an expert at cooking, it's a stir-fry. It's quick, easy, tasty, nutritious and low in calories. By learning just one recipe, you will be able to cook 10 or more meals by substituting different protein (kangaroo, chicken, fish, tofu) and vegetables.

Heat half the oil in a non-stick wok on high. Stir-fry the beef in 2 batches for 1 minute until browned. Set aside.

Heat the remaining oil in the wok on high. Stir-fry the green beans for 3 minutes. Add the zucchini and stir-fry for another 3 minutes until just tender.

Return the beef to the wok with the garlic, ginger, sauces and gai larn. Stir-fry for another minute until the gai larn starts to wilt. Serve immediately.

Tip
- Hoisin sauce can be salty and sugary, so pick one that has around 200 mg of sodium and 20 calories for every 20 ml (tablespoon).

Variation
- Serve with rice for a heartier family meal.

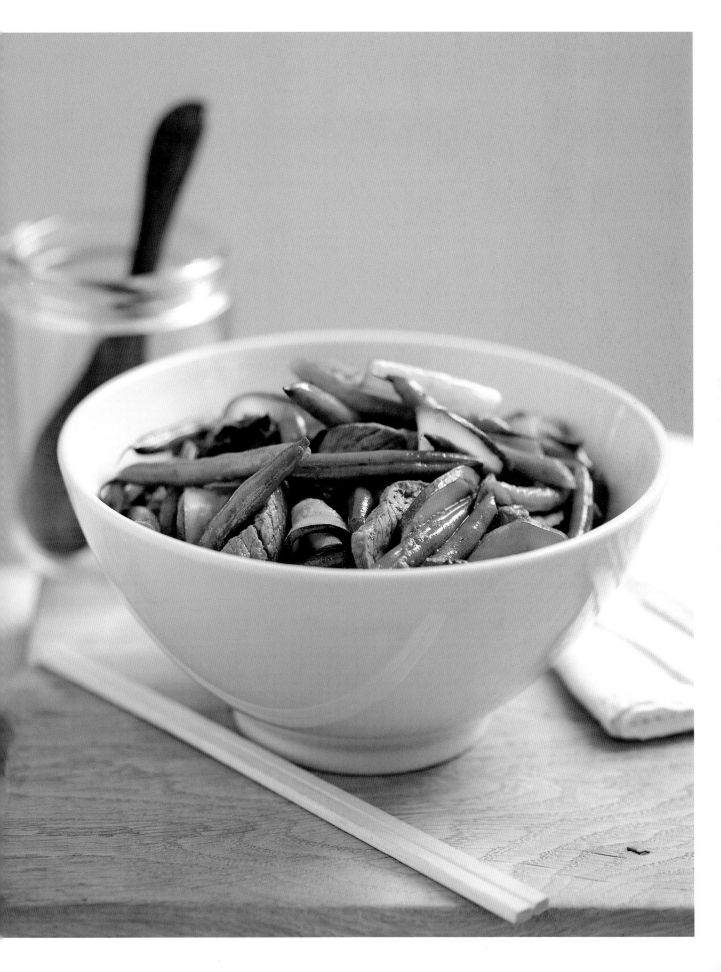

Chilli beef stir-fry

Serves 2
Prep 15 minutes
Cook 10 minutes
323 cal per serve

---

2 teaspoons vegetable oil
220 g rump steak, trimmed
    and cut into strips
1 large onion, halved and cut
    into wedges
2 medium carrots, cut into batons
1 yellow capsicum, cut into batons
1 bunch spinach, washed,
    trimmed and coarsely chopped
2 teaspoons freshly grated ginger
2 teaspoons chilli garlic sauce
1 tablespoon tamari
1 long red chilli, thinly sliced on
    the diagonal
⅓ cup coriander leaves, to serve

This stir-fry makes me feel like a master in the kitchen! I've used tamari, the Japanese version of soy sauce, but you can use salt-reduced soy if you prefer. With stir-fries it doesn't really matter if you don't have all the spices or sauces – they'll still taste delicious because the light cooking style means the vegies burst with flavour.

Heat half the oil in a non-stick wok on high. Stir-fry the beef in 2 batches for 1 minute until browned. Set aside.

Heat the remaining oil in the wok on high. Stir-fry the onion, carrot and capsicum for 3–4 minutes until just tender. Return the beef to the wok with the spinach, ginger, sauces, chilli and 1 tablespoon water. Stir-fry for 1 minute until the spinach is just wilted.

Serve immediately, garnished with coriander.

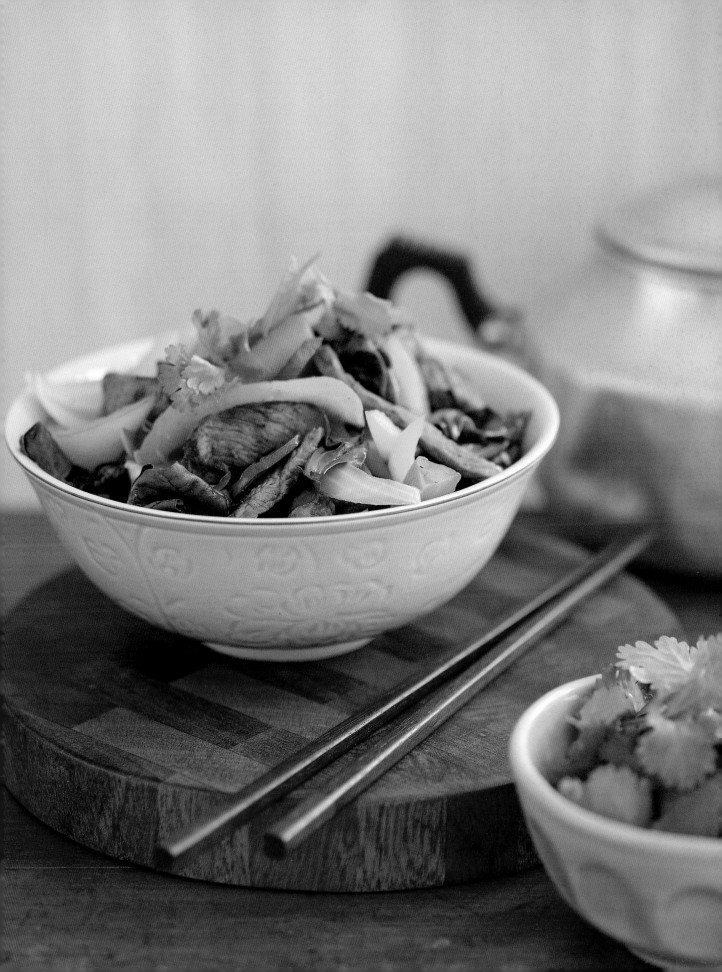

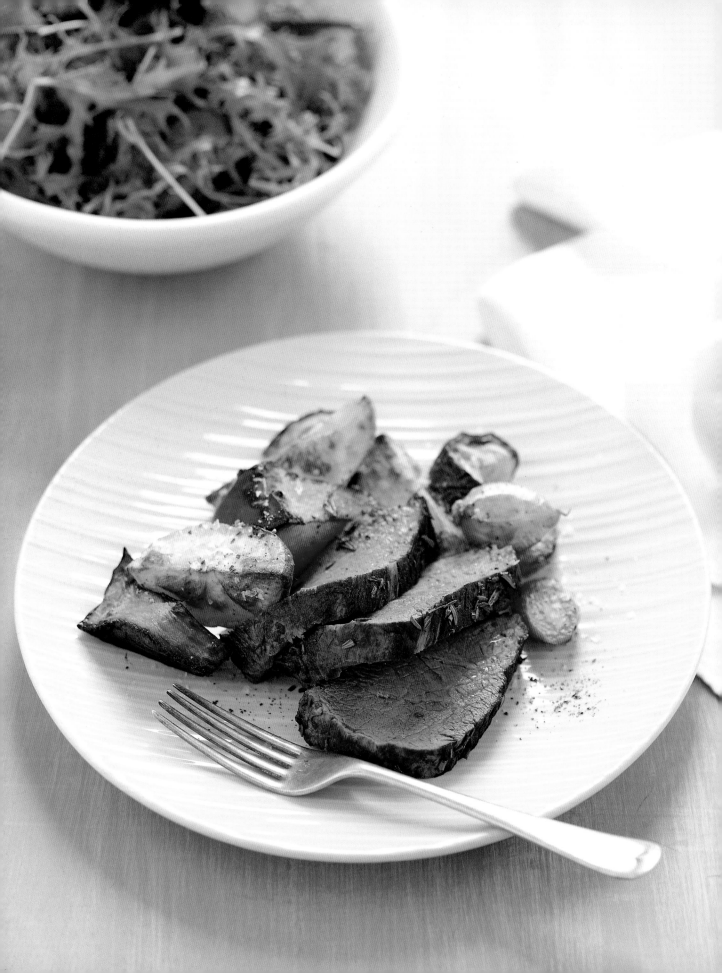

Roast beef and vegetables

I cook this for my mum and she loves it! Remember that you can substitute whatever vegetables you happen to have in the fridge. Baked parsnip is a personal favourite, but try pumpkin, sweet potato or swede. I've used beef fillet here as it's very lean – but it is expensive. Sirloin is slightly cheaper and a rolled rib is probably the most cost effective, though it is fattier. Allow around 180 g per person (220 g if the meat is on the bone). Of course it goes without saying that leftover beef is great for sandwiches (see page 81).

Preheat the oven to 230°C. Place the vegetables and garlic in a large roasting pan. Lightly spray with olive oil and season to taste with pepper. Roast for 30 minutes.

Meanwhile, rub the beef with the olive oil and rosemary, and a little pepper. Lightly spray a frying pan with oil and heat on high. Sear the beef on each side until browned. Remove the roasting pan from the oven and make a space in the centre of the vegetables. Transfer the beef to the roasting pan and roast for 25 minutes for rare or 35 minutes for medium–rare.

Cover the beef loosely with foil and rest in a warm place for 10 minutes before slicing. Serve with the roasted vegetables and salad.

Tip
- For fewer calories, instead of potato use 400 g peeled sweet potato cut into chunks (292 calories per serve).

Serves 8
Prep 15 minutes
Cook 1 hour
309 cal per serve

600 g Kent pumpkin, unpeeled and cut into chunks
4 medium potatoes, unpeeled and quartered lengthways
2 large zucchini, cut into chunks
2 large carrots, cut into chunks
8 garlic cloves, unpeeled
olive oil spray
freshly ground black pepper
1.2 kg beef fillet, at room temperature
2 teaspoons olive oil
2 teaspoons coarsely chopped rosemary
120 g mixed salad leaves, to serve

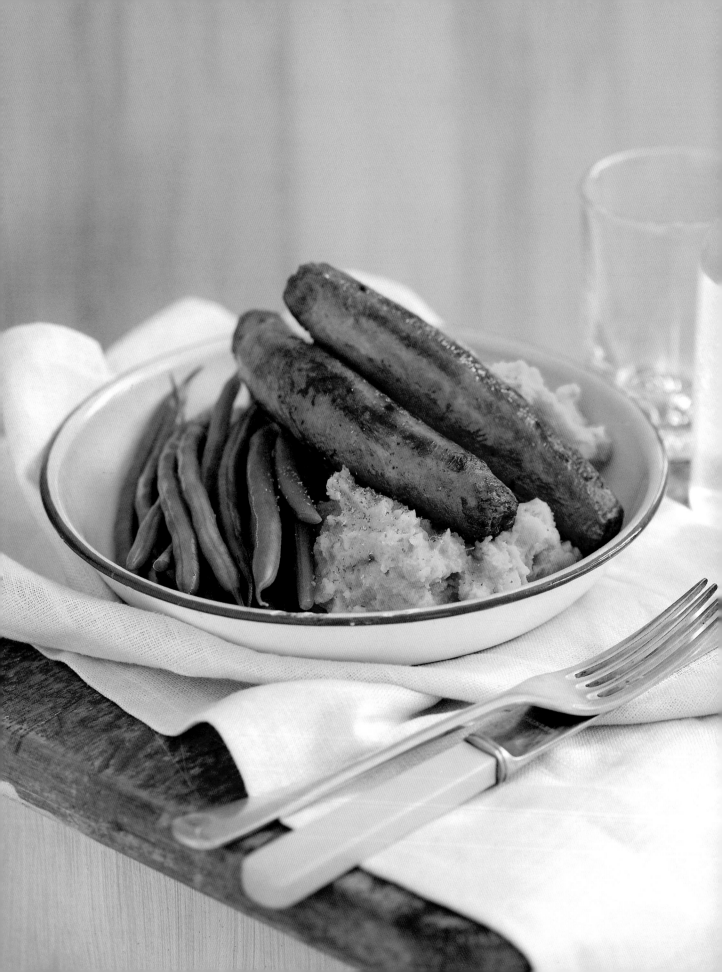

Kanga Bangas with sweet potato mash

I was so happy when I discovered these kangaroo sausages! Now I can have snags at my summer barbies without the fat and calories. Kanga Bangas are super low in fat and calories (50 calories each!) and really high in protein. I often cook up a few extra and have them cold on a sandwich or as a snack the next day.

To make the mash, place the sweet potato and garlic in a small saucepan. Cover with water and bring to the boil. Simmer, covered, for 10 minutes until tender. Drain. Mash, then mix in the milk until combined. Season with pepper and nutmeg.

Meanwhile, lightly spray a non-stick frying pan with olive oil and heat on medium. Cook the sausages for 8 minutes, turning regularly, until browned and cooked through.

Serve the sausages with the sweet potato mash and steamed green beans.

Variation
- I like to keep my calories tight at night so I will often just have my bangers with 200 g steamed greens (210 calories).
- Try a **cauliflower and parsnip mash** – it's a great alternative and really keeps the GI low. Simply steam the florets from ¼ head cauliflower with 1 chopped parsnip until they are very soft, add a dollop of low-cal ricotta and mash by hand (or use a blender if you like your mash very creamy). For an extra kick, add a smear of wasabi.

Serves 2
Prep 10 minutes
Cook 10 minutes
347 cal per serve

olive oil spray
4 × 75 g kangaroo sausages
　(Kanga Bangas)
200 g steamed green beans,
　to serve

sweet potato mash
450 g sweet potato, peeled
　and cut into chunks
1 garlic clove
½ cup skim milk
freshly ground black pepper
pinch freshly grated nutmeg

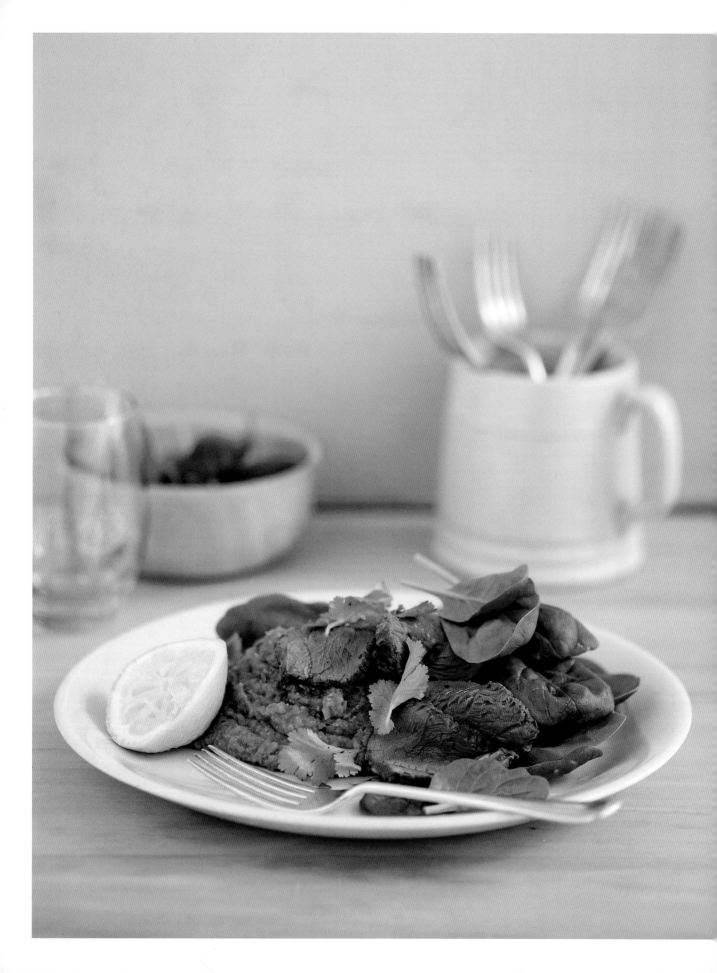

Roast kangaroo with lentil and cumin mash

This meal is super-versatile and delicious. Make plenty of it – it keeps well and makes great sandwiches. When reheating, stir in a little vegetable stock as the mash can dry out a bit in the fridge.

Preheat the oven to 220°C. Without removing the string, pat dry the roast with paper towel. Lightly spray an ovenproof non-stick frying pan with olive oil and heat on medium–high. Sear the roast on each side until browned. Transfer the pan to the oven and roast the kangaroo for 18 minutes for rare. (If you don't have an ovenproof frying pan, transfer the roast to a roasting pan or baking dish.)

Meanwhile, make the mash. Lightly spray a medium saucepan with oil and heat on medium. Cook the onion and garlic for 5 minutes, stirring, until softened. Stir in the cumin and cook for 1 minute until fragrant. Add the lentils and ¾ cup water. Reduce the heat to low and cook, covered, for 10 minutes.

Remove the roast from the pan and stand, loosely covered, for 5 minutes. Meanwhile, using a hand-held blender, coarsely puree the lentils. Add the lemon juice and chopped coriander and season to taste with pepper.

Slice half of the roast. (Set aside the remaining half for another meal.) Serve the roast with the lentil mash and the baby spinach. Garnish the mash with the coriander sprigs.

Tip
- Herb and garlic kangaroo roasts are produced by Macro Meats and can be found in supermarkets.

Variations
- I prefer to use dried lentils. Just follow the directions on the packet for soaking or rapid boiling. You'll need about 1 cup of dried lentils to make an amount equivalent to two cans.
- The mash is also great with other meats, such as beef or lamb. Try it with roast beef (see page 181) instead of baked vegies.

Serves 4
Prep 10 minutes
Cook 20 minutes
317 cal per serve

1 × 525 g herb and garlic kangaroo roast (see below)
olive oil spray
3 handfuls baby spinach, to serve

lentil and cumin mash
1 onion, finely chopped
2 garlic cloves
½ teaspoon cumin seeds
2 × 400 g cans red or yellow lentils, drained, rinsed
½ lemon, juice only
⅓ cup freshly chopped coriander, plus extra sprigs to garnish
freshly ground black pepper

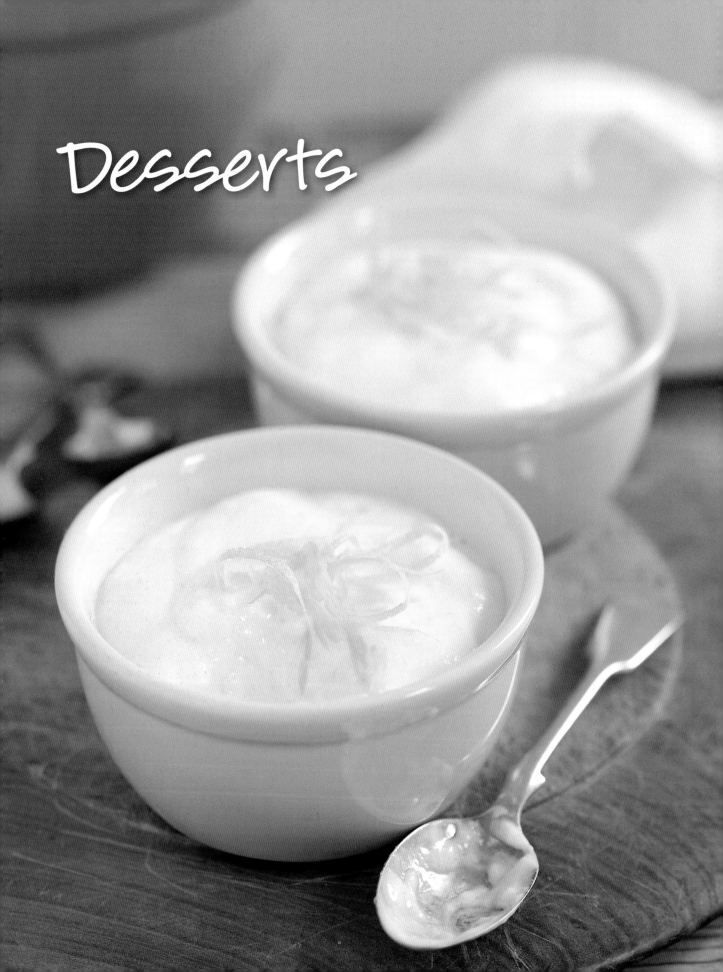

Desserts

Lemon mousse

This little gem has it all – lots of fruit, protein from the egg whites, and served in a measured portion. And did I mention that it tastes fantastic? Try it with lime instead of lemon.

Serves 6
Prep 15 minutes
Chill 2–3 hours
102 cal per serve

⅓ cup low-GI sugar
2 tablespoons boiling water
2 teaspoons powdered gelatine
2 egg whites
1½ cups low-cal plain yoghurt
½ lemon, juice and zest, plus
   extra zest to decorate
100 g raspberries, to serve

Using a small blender or a pestle and mortar, grind the low-GI sugar to a fine powder. Combine the water and gelatine in a small jug and stir until dissolved.

Using an electric mixer, beat the egg whites until soft peaks form. Gradually add the ground sugar, beating until thick and glossy.

Combine the yoghurt, zest and juice in a bowl. Whisk in the gelatine mixture, then fold in the egg-white mixture until combined. Spoon into 6 glasses, then cover and refrigerate for 2–3 hours until set. Decorate the mousse with the extra zest and serve with the raspberries.

Poached rhubarb with yoghurt and basil

Serves 8
Prep 5 minutes
Cook 10 minutes
103 cal per serve

⅓ cup low-GI sugar
juice of 1 orange
500 g rhubarb, cut into 4 cm pieces
750 g low-cal plain yoghurt
2 tablespoons freshly shredded basil leaves

Rhubarb doesn't get used in cooking as much as it did in our grandmothers' day, but its tart flavour is great when sweetened. Here I use it as a garnish for yoghurt, which makes for a nutritious low-calorie dessert.

Place the sugar and orange juice in a medium saucepan. Stir over a low heat until the sugar has dissolved, then bring to the boil. Add the rhubarb and reduce the heat to low. Cook, covered, for 8–10 minutes until the rhubarb is soft but still holds its shape. Cool in the pan.

To serve, divide the yoghurt among 8 shallow bowls and top with poached rhubarb. Sprinkle with basil.

Tips
- Never eat the leaves of rhubarb – they are toxic.
- This serves 8, so unless you have a family (or guests for dinner) put 6 serves away for breakfasts (see page 51) or freezing.
- If you're using the poached rhubarb for breakfast or for another recipe, note that the total calories are 424.

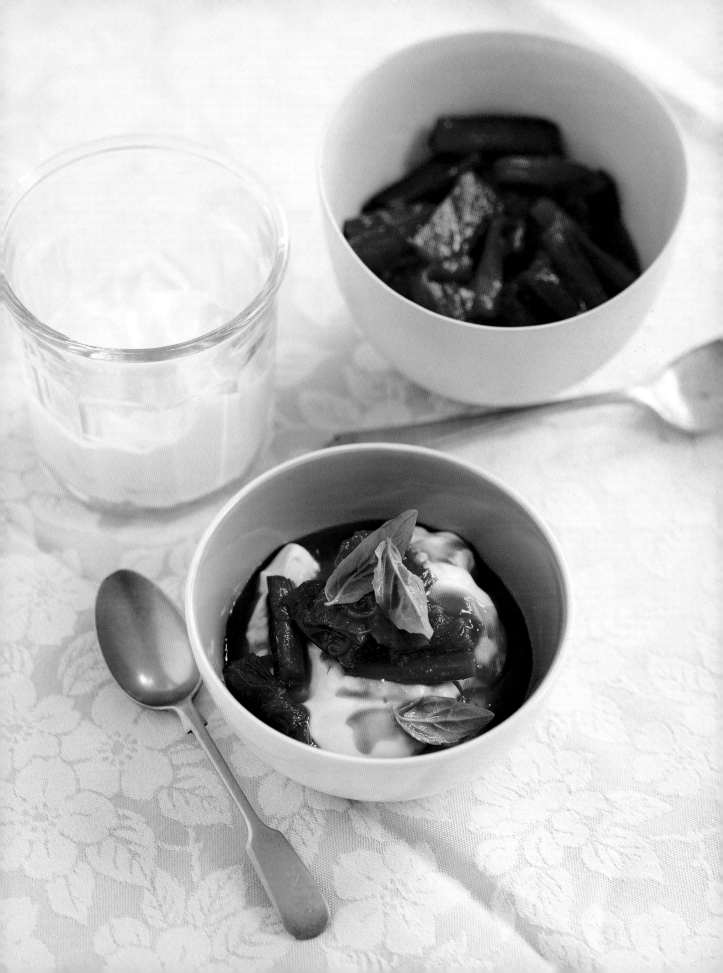

Strawberry and passionfruit yoghurt semifreddo

Serves 10
Prep 20 minutes
Freeze overnight
103 cal per serve

2 tablespoons passionfruit pulp
300 g strawberries
1 tablespoon icing sugar, sifted
¼ cup low-GI sugar
3 eggs
560 g low-cal vanilla yoghurt

This looks divine and is packed with good ingredients like low-fat yoghurt, strawberries and passionfruit. If you've got friends coming over and you're planning a bit of an occasion, it can be handy to prepare some of the food the day before. This is one of the reasons why semifreddo is a good dinner party dessert choice. Don't forget to get it out of the freezer 20 minutes or so before serving, though.

Line the long sides of a 6-cup loaf pan with plastic wrap, leaving enough hanging over the sides to fold over and enclose the semifreddo. Spread the passionfruit pulp over the base.

Hull 200 g of the strawberries and coarsely puree them with a fork. Stir in the icing sugar until combined.

Using a small blender or a pestle and mortar, grind the low-GI sugar to a fine powder. Using an electric mixer, beat the eggs and ground sugar for 5 minutes until pale and thick. Gently stir through the yoghurt. Pour into the prepared pan. Gently spoon over dollops of the strawberry mixture (it will sink slightly). Fold over and enclose with the plastic wrap and freeze overnight.

Next day, transfer the semifreddo to the main part of the fridge 20 minutes before serving to soften slightly. Unfold the plastic wrap and turn the semifreddo out onto a plate. Remove the plastic wrap. Cut the semifreddo into slices and divide among the serving plates. Serve with the remaining strawberries.

Tips
• Low-GI sugar has large granules, so you need to grind it to make it fine enough to mix with the eggs.
• If you have fewer than 10 people at your dinner party, freeze the rest in individual portions for another special occasion.

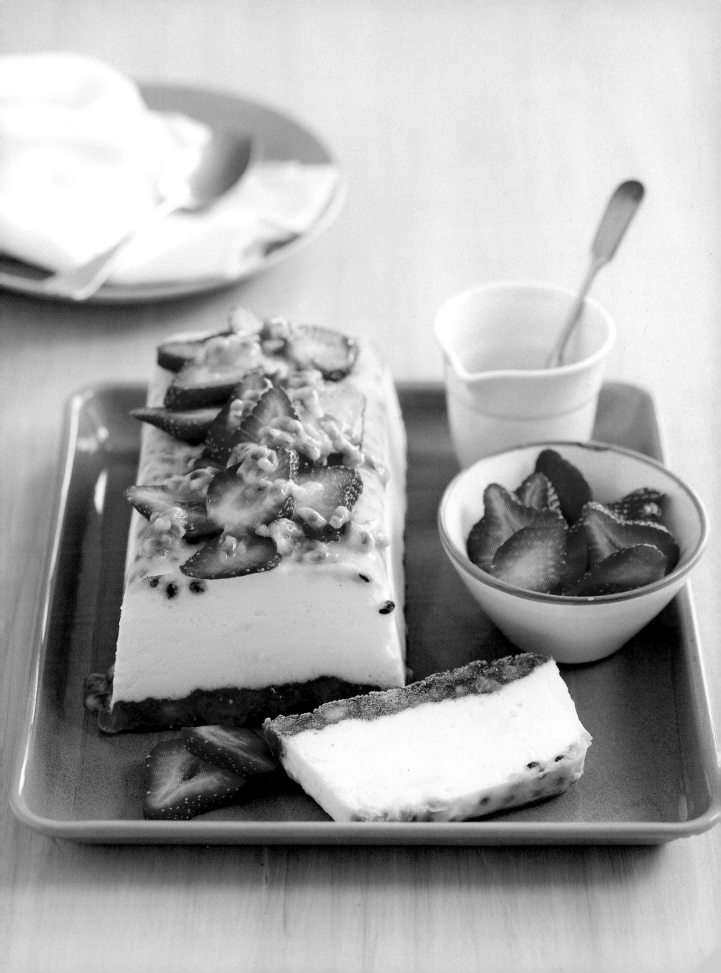

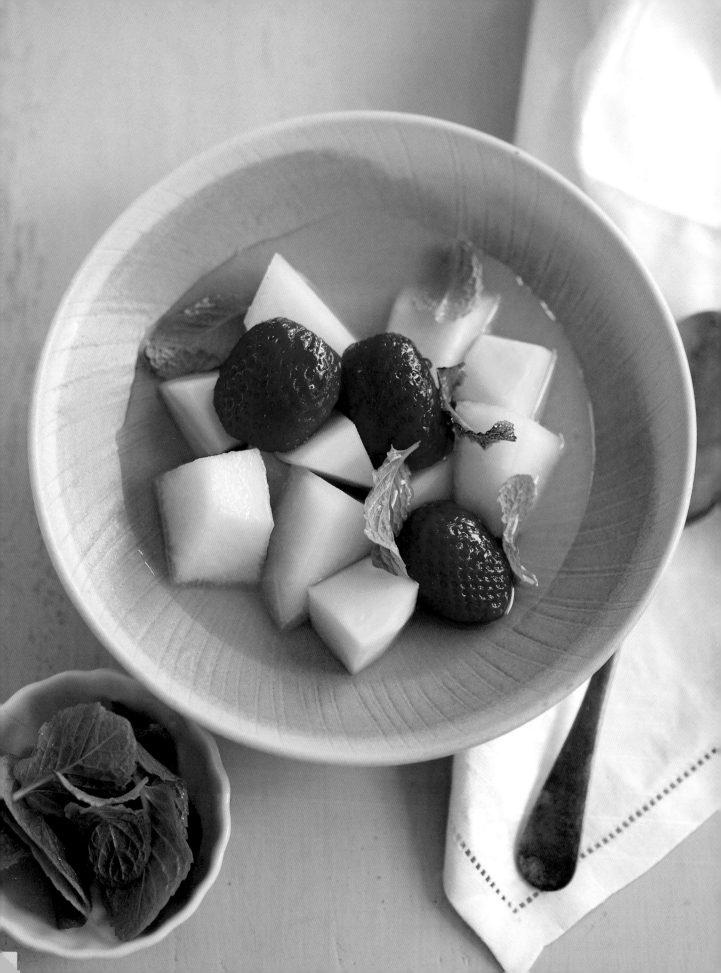

Ginger and lime fruit salad

How could a recipe with a name like this be anything but delicious? Mango, melon, ginger and strawberries and still only 100 or so calories a serve!

Removed the lime zest in strips with a vegetable peeler, and squeeze the juice. In a small heavy saucepan, combine the zest, ⅓ cup lime juice, the sugar, the ginger and ⅓ cup water. Heat gently, stirring, until the sugar has dissolved. Bring to the boil and cook for 5 minutes. Pour the syrup through a fine sieve into a bowl and let it cool.

Combine the fruit in a serving bowl. Add the syrup and toss to coat. Refrigerate, covered, for 2 hours or overnight. Stir through the mint before serving.

Serves 8
Prep 15 minutes
Cook 5 minutes
Chill 2 hours
110 cal per serve

1 lime
¼ cup low-GI sugar
1 tablespoon freshly grated ginger
1 honeydew melon, seeded and cut into cubes
1 mango, flesh cut into cubes
500 g strawberries
¼ cup fresh mint leaves

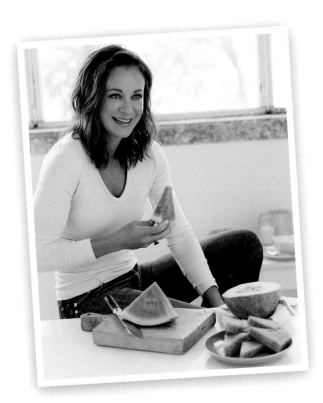

Berry jelly

Makes 8
Prep 20 minutes
Cook 5 minutes
Chill 3 hours
99 cal per serve

1½ cups white wine
1½ cups cranberry juice
¼ cup low-GI sugar
1 tablespoon powdered gelatine
500 g fresh mixed berries
  (strawberries, raspberries,
  blueberries, blackberries)

This recipe might seem a little more fiddly than the others, but don't be put off. It's fun to make, the kids will enjoy helping (just use juice instead of wine for their version), and of course it tastes great with all the mixed berries. I also like how it is served in measured portions, which reduces the risk of spooning a big portion into your bowl.

Place the wine, juice and sugar in a saucepan and stir over a low heat for 3 minutes until the sugar has dissolved. Sprinkle in the gelatine and stir to dissolve thoroughly. Set aside to cool completely without setting.

Meanwhile, cut the berries into bite-sized pieces. Set aside 200 g berries. Moisten 8 × ½ cup dariole moulds or glasses and pour about 5 mm of jelly mixture into each one. Refrigerate for 10–15 minutes until sticky. Scatter a little fruit over the layer of jelly and carefully pour over a little more wine mixture to just cover the fruit. Return to the refrigerator for 10–15 minutes until sticky. Continue making layers of fruit and jelly this way until all the wine jelly mixture has been used and the moulds are full. Refrigerate for 3 hours until very firm and set.

To serve, dip the base of each mould into a bowl of very hot water for a second only, then carefully invert the jelly onto a serving plate. Serve with the remaining berries.

Tip
• If the jelly does not slip out, give the mould a sharp shake to help release it.

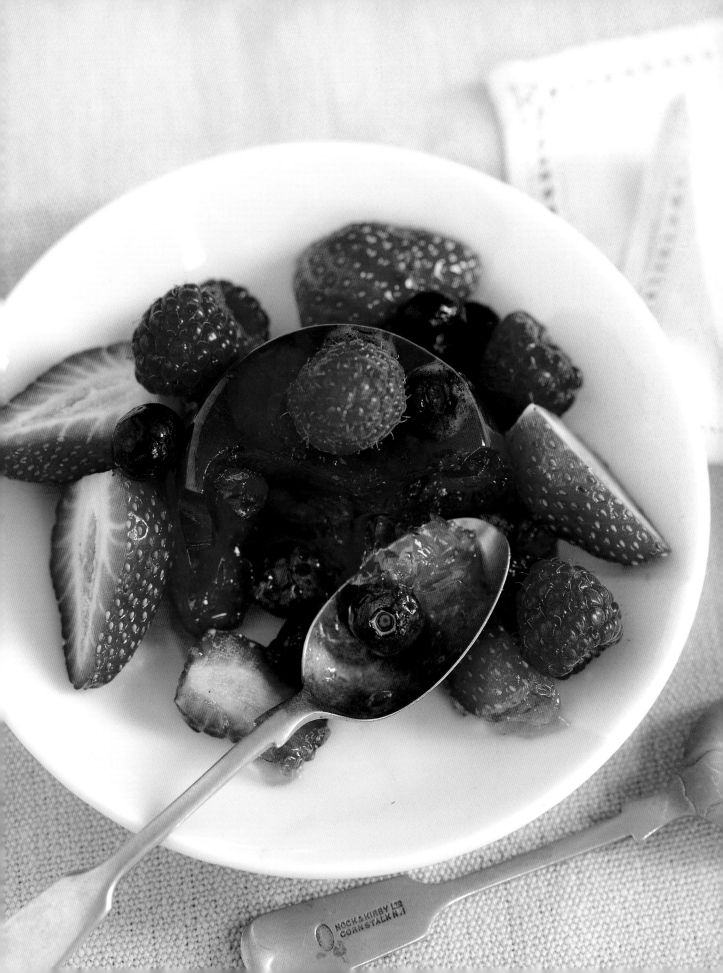

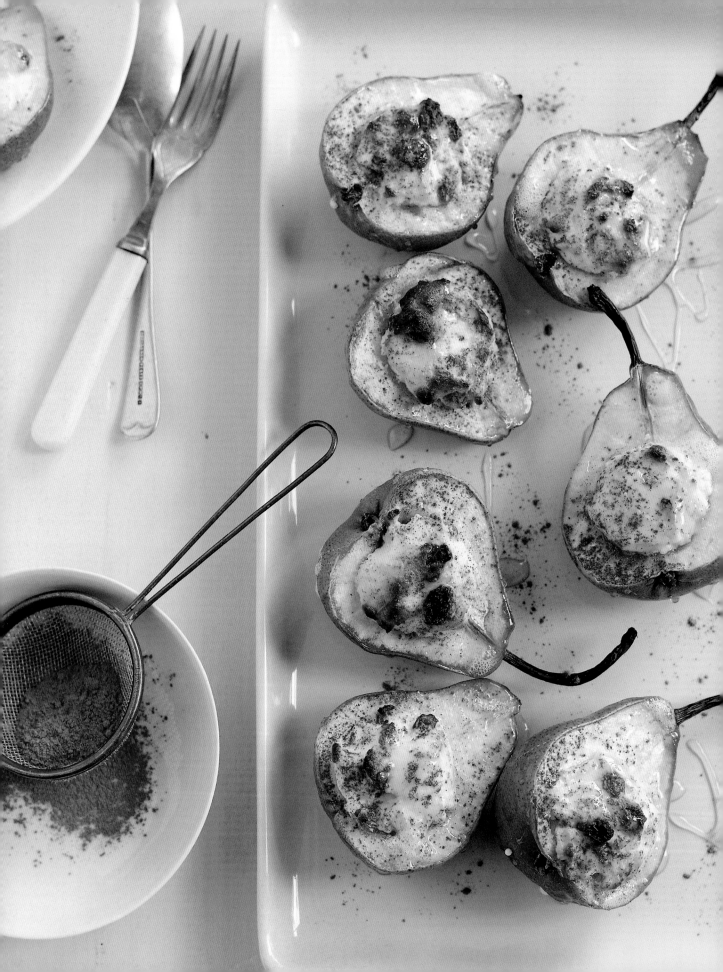

Baked pears and ricotta with honey, sultanas and cinnamon

This dish is a cracker for saving time and money. It's also really delicious.

Preheat the oven to 180°C. Line a baking sheet with baking paper.

Using a teaspoon, scoop out the seeds and core of each pear half to make a round hollow. Place the pear halves on the prepared baking sheet. Combine the ricotta and sultanas in a small bowl, then spoon into the pear hollows. Drizzle with honey and sprinkle with cinnamon.

Bake for 30 minutes until the pears are tender. Cool a little before serving.

Tip

• If you're having people around for dinner and you're roasting meat or vegetables, pop the pears into the oven at the same time as your roast.

Serves 8
Prep 10 minutes
Cook 30 minutes
107 cal per serve

4 large, firm ripe pears, halved with stems intact
150 g low-cal ricotta
2 tablespoons sultanas, chopped
1 tablespoon honey
ground cinnamon

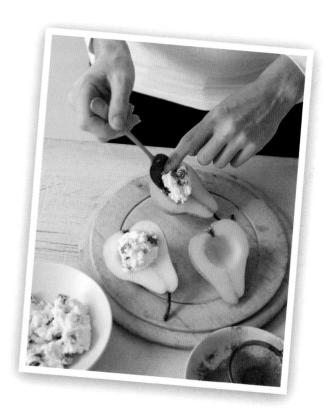

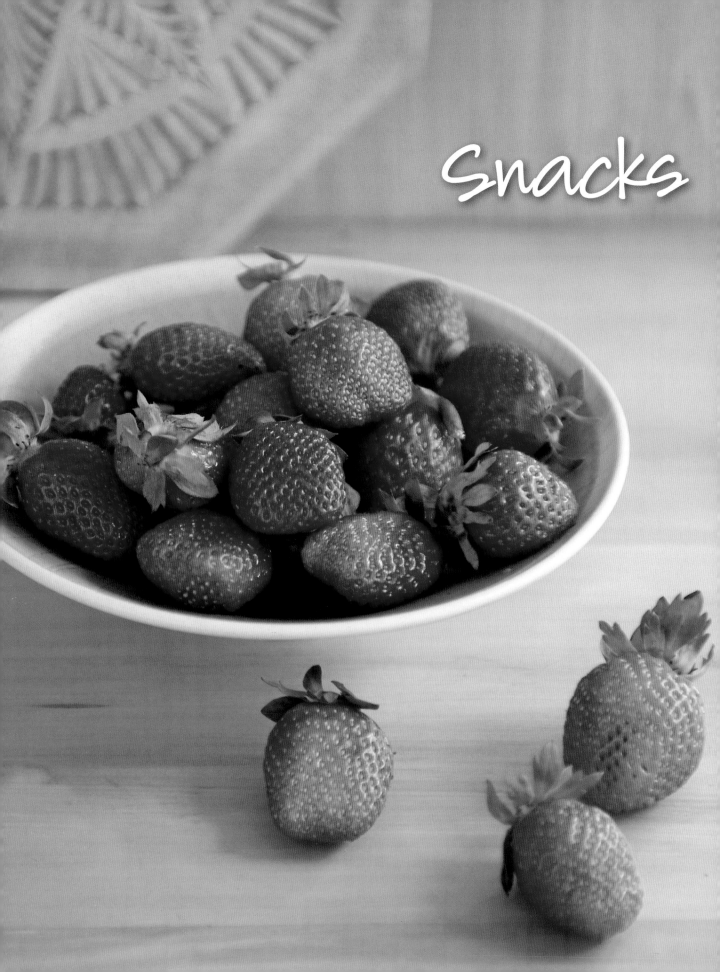

Snacks

Snacks are handy when you know you won't be eating lunch or dinner until late, or when you have a big training session coming up. The whole idea of a snack is convenience. It should be quick, easy, healthy and never more than 100–150 calories. Some of my snacks are supremely simple, like a medium apple (75 calories), a banana (80 calories), a tub of low-cal yoghurt (81 calories) or a big handful of strawberries (40 calories). Others require very little time to make, and a couple can be made on the weekend to provide you with a week's worth of snacks. It's all about being organised so that you have the snack with you and are not tempted to grab something salty, sugary and over packaged.

Pear and cottage crackers

All good snacks need to be quick and this one is just that: two multigrain Vitawheats topped with some thinly sliced pear and a dollop of low-fat cottage cheese. Yum!

Around 113 calories

Cottage sticks

Celery is such an awesome vegetable, super delicious and super crunchy. Top three big sticks with some low-fat cottage cheese and dot a few sultanas along the top.

Around 131 calories

Cherry ripe

Okay, it's not the one you might be thinking of. This is my version! A low-fat, low-calorie hot chocolate while munching on 10 fresh cherries! Delicious! Make your hot chocolate with skim milk or half skim milk, half hot water.

Around 114 calories

Italian tomato

This is definitely a favourite of mine! Three large slices of tomato, topped with a slice of bocconcini and finished with a large basil leaf. Not only are they quick to do but they look really lovely, too.

Around 71 calories

Very berry

Berries are the bomb when it comes to antioxidants, plus they are super-low in calories and downright yummy! One cup of fresh strawberries and half a cup of fresh blueberries, one dollop of low-cal yoghurt on top and you are good to go.

Around 99 calories

Fruit bread

I like this one because it's quick and delicious, but make sure you put the rest of the loaf away immediately. One slice of low GI fruit bread fresh or toasted, smeared with low-cal cream cheese or cottage cheese.

Around 104 calories

Hummus

Makes 2½ cups
Prep 10 minutes
Cook 40 minutes
Stand overnight
100 cal per serve (3 tablespoons
   plus vegies)

---

1 cup dried chickpeas
1 onion, peeled but left whole
1 bay leaf
2 tablespoons tahini
2 garlic cloves, crushed
2 tablespoons lemon juice
1 tablespoon extra virgin olive oil
freshly ground black pepper
100 g fresh vegetable sticks
   per serve (e.g. carrot, celery,
   zucchini)

This creamy spread made from chickpeas is a favourite in Australian kitchens, and it's easy to see why. It's perfect as a dip with raw vegetables, and as a spread in sandwiches and wraps. Tahini is sesame seed paste and is easy to find in any supermarket. Be careful that you don't go overboard with hummus, though; it's 70 calories for 3 tablespoons.

Soak the chick peas in water overnight. Drain.

Place the chickpeas in a large saucepan with the onion and bay leaf. Cover with water and bring to the boil. Simmer for 40 minutes until the chickpeas are tender. Remove and discard the onion and bay leaf. Drain the chickpeas, reserving ⅔ cup cooking liquid.

Combine the chickpeas, tahini, garlic, lemon juice and reserved cooking liquid in a bowl. Using a hand-held blender, puree until smooth (or leave slightly chunky if you prefer). Stir in the olive oil and season to taste with pepper.

Serve with the vegetable sticks.

Tips

- If you are in a hurry, use a 400 g can of chickpeas instead.
- Use the same method to cook other pulses, such as lentils or split peas (the cooking time may vary). Never add salt to pulses when cooking – they won't soften.

Bruschetta

Traditional Italian bruschetta is simply toasted bread rubbed with garlic and moistened with a little olive oil, but there are lots of different toppings you can add. See what you have in the fridge and don't be scared to experiment with different combinations! I don't put oil on my bruschetta, but if you must use it, a couple of drops is all you need.

Mix the tomato, red onion and basil in a small bowl. Toast or grill the breadstick slices, then rub one side with the garlic clove. Top with the tomato mixture and season with pepper.

Variations

- Other toppings to try: hummus (see opposite) and baby spinach leaves; orange segments (pith removed) and finely sliced fennel; char-grilled eggplant (see page 78) and low-cal ricotta; or char-grilled capsicum (see page 106) and freshly chopped thyme.

Serves 2
Prep 10 minutes
108 cal

½ cup diced fresh tomato
¼ cup finely diced red onion
¼ cup freshly shredded basil
2 slices breadstick
1 garlic clove
freshly ground black pepper

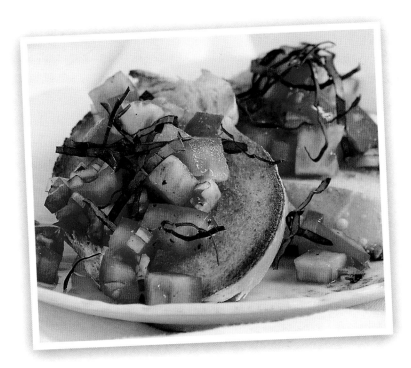

Tzatziki

Makes 2 cups
Prep 10 minutes
100 cal per serve (including vegies)

---

2 Lebanese cucumbers, grated
400 g Greek-style low-cal yoghurt
2 garlic cloves, crushed
¼ cup freshly chopped mint
1 tablespoon lemon juice
pinch salt and freshly ground
  black pepper
120 g fresh vegetable sticks
  per serve (e.g. carrot, celery,
  zucchini)

I love this tangy, refreshing dip. It goes well with the mild flavours of many vegetables, tastes fantastic with grilled lamb, and is great in sandwiches too. I've calculated one serve as ¼ cup (3 level tablespoons), which is around 70 calories.

Place the cucumber in a fine sieve and press down to remove any liquid. Combine the cucumber, yoghurt, garlic, mint and lemon juice in a bowl. Season to taste with salt and pepper. Serve with the vegetable sticks.

Tips

● I've included this recipe more for using on sandwiches than having as a snack, but it's great to serve to guests on special occasions.

● Make a quick summer soup by adding cold water to the tzatziki.

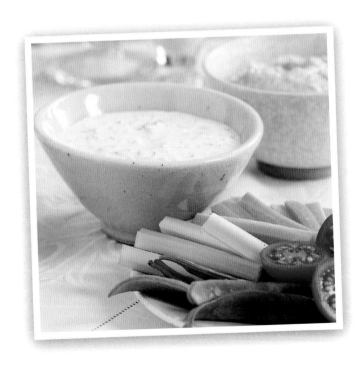

Apricot and buttermilk muffins

These muffins are yummy – but remember that they are rather high in calories. I like to use rice bran oil, which is rich in vitamin E and 'healthier' than many other oils. It should be available at your supermarket. Buttermilk gives a lighter texture to muffins than regular milk. It is also available at the supermarket, but if you can't find it, use skim milk.

Preheat the oven to 200°C. Line a 12-hole muffin pan with paper cases.

Combine the flour, sugar and apricots in a bowl. In another bowl, whisk together the buttermilk, egg, oil and lemon zest. Add the wet ingredients to the flour mixture and stir until just combined. The batter will still be lumpy.

Spoon the batter into the prepared pan. Bake for 18 minutes or until golden and a skewer comes out clean.

Tips

• Muffins are great in school lunch boxes, but if you're trying to lose weight, keep them for a rare treat.

• Wrap individual muffins in aluminium foil and freeze them for later use.

Makes 12
Prep 10 minutes
Cook 20 minutes
151 cal per muffin

1¾ cups self-raising flour
1 tablespoon low-GI sugar
⅓ cup chopped dried apricots
1 cup buttermilk
1 small egg
¼ cup rice bran oil
1 lemon, zest only

Olive and basil muffins

Makes 12
Prep 10 minutes
Cook 20 minutes
147 cal per muffin

1¾ cups wholemeal self-raising
   flour
⅓ cup grated parmesan
220 ml skim milk
1 medium egg
¼ cup olive oil
50 g olives, pitted and chopped
¼ cup freshly chopped basil

Muffins are really easy to make, but be aware that if you eat more than one, you'll blow your daily calorie quota (two muffins will give you a similar calorie load to your main meal). Enjoy them only very occasionally!

Preheat the oven to 200°C. Line a 12-hole muffin pan with paper cases.

Combine the flour and parmesan in a large bowl. Combine the milk, egg and oil in another bowl, then stir through the olives and basil. Add the wet ingredients to the flour mixture and stir until just combined. The batter will still be lumpy.

Spoon the batter into the prepared pan. Bake for 18 minutes or until golden and a skewer comes out clean.

Tip

● Wrap individual muffins in aluminium foil and freeze them for later use.

Berry smoothie

Everyone loves a delicious fruit smoothie, and it's a good option for a healthy snack. I love it with fresh strawberries, but you can try it with any kind of berry or a mixture of berries. In summer, use frozen berries to make a gorgeous frappe.

Combine all the ingredients in a blender. Serve immediately.

Variations

• Try blueberries, raspberries or blackberries instead of strawberries, or a combination of berries.
• Drop the honey to reduce the calorie count by 20.
• Use half skim milk and half water to get the calories down to only 86.
• Try a sprinkling of unsugared ground cinnamon or a drop of vanilla essence for a more delicate flavour.

Makes 1
Prep 5 minutes
154 cal

½ cup strawberries, halved
1 cup skim milk
2 tablespoons low-cal plain yoghurt
1 teaspoon honey

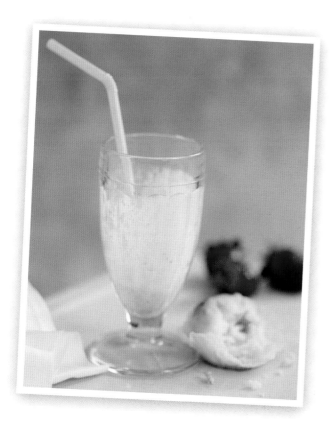

Index

C

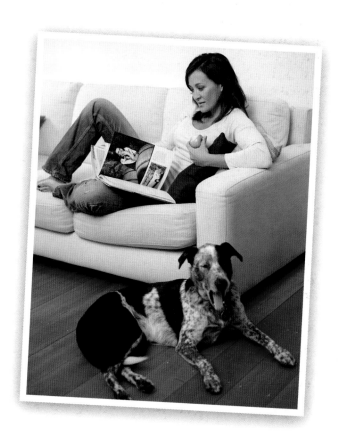

Acknowledgements

I would like to thank all the people who supported my first book, *Crunch Time*, as its success inspired this one. Cooking has become such a passion of mine over the years. Nothing brings people together like food, and it is my dream to have more Australian families cooking for each other and enjoying the benefits of healthy nutrition in their homes.

There are many people I need to thank for *Crunch Time Cookbook*. Thanks to my beloved husband, Billy, my MasterChef! Without you many of these recipes would not have been created. To my mum, for teaching me the importance of good nutrition at home. To the team at Penguin, who believed in this project: Kirsten Abbott, Miriam Cannell, Cameron Midson, Felicity Vallence, Dan Ruffino and Sally Bateman. To the talented Lucy Nunes, my wonderful recipe designer.

To my amazing team at Chic Celebrity Management: Ursula Hufnagl, Jane Weston, Wendy Wilson and Theo Chryssan, who just get it done. To Carl Fennessy and the wonderful team at Fremantle Media. To Dafydd Williams, David Mott and the fabulous gang at Channel Ten, all of whom have really believed in my message. To my wonderful sponsor Adidas. To Louise Keats, her mum Suzanne Gibbs and her mum Margaret Fulton, who all showed me the beautiful and wonderful world of home cooking. The photographic team of Mark O'Meara and Nick Wilson, and the foodie team Michelle Noerianto and Jennifer Tolhurst. To Wayne Chick, who made me look fab. To the gang at About Life in Rozelle, who allowed us to use their fabulous supermarket. To Loo and Ann from Baffi & Mo café. And of course to all those people who bought *Crunch Time* and changed their lives for the better! Thank you!